RACE
& RESEARCH

Perspectives on
Minority Participation
in Health Studies

Edited By: Bettina M. Beech, DrPH and Maurine Goodman, MA, MPH

APHA
American Public Health Association

American Public Health Association
800 I Street, NW
Washington, DC 20001
www.apha.org

Georges Benjamin, MD, FACP, Executive Director
Carolyn K. Mikanowicz, PhD, APHA Publications Board Liaison

Printed and bound in the United States of America
Typesetting: Susan Westrate
Cover Design: Michele Pryor
Set in: Goudy and Univers
Printing and Binding: Kirby Lithographic Co., Inc.

ISBN: 0-87553-030-3

2.5 M 2/04

NOTE: Any discussion of medical or legal issues in this publication is being provided for informational purposes only. Nothing in this publication is intended to constitute medical or legal advice, and it should not be construed as such. This book is not intended to be and should not be used as a substitute for specific medical or legal advice, since medical and legal opinions may only be given in response to inquiries regarding specific factual situations. If medical or legal advice is desired by the reader of this book, a medical doctor or attorney should be consulted.

The use of trade names and commercial sources in this book does not imply endorsement by either the APHA or the editorial board of this volume.

TABLE *of* CONTENTS

Section III
Evolutionary Changes in Medicine and Health Care

CONTRIBUTORS

Collins O. Airhihenbuwa, PhD, MPH
The Pennsylvania State University
Department of Biobehavioral Health
College of Health and Human Development
University Park, PA

Bettina M. Beech, DrPH, MPH
University of Memphis
Department of Psychology
Memphis, TN

Derrick J. Beech, MD, FACS
University of Tennessee Health Science
 Center
Department of Surgery, Surgical Oncology
Memphis, TN

David Blumenthal, MD, PhD
Institute for Health Policy
Harvard University
Boston, MA

Eric G. Campbell, PhD
Institute for Health Policy
Harvard University
Boston, MA

Susan D. Cochran, PhD, MS
UCLA School of Public Health
Los Angeles, CA

Elizabeth Fore, MEd
University of South Carolina
Norman J. Arnold School of Public Health
Department of Health Promotion and
 Education and Women's Studies Program
Columbia, SC

Morris W. Foster, PhD
Department of Anthropology
University of Oklahoma
Norman, OK
Arthritis and Immunology Program
Oklahoma Medical Research Foundation
Oklahoma City, OK

Tiffany L. Gary, PhD
Welch Center for Prevention Epidemiology,
 and Clinical Research
Johns Hopkins Medical Institutions
Department of Epidemiology
Johns Hopkins Bloomberg School of Public
 Health
Baltimore, MD

Maurine Goodman, MA, MPH
Department of Community Health Sciences
School of Public Health
Tulane University
New Orleans, LA

Elizabeth Heitman, PhD
Associate Professor
University of Texas–Houston
School of Public Health
Houston, TX

Leonard Jack, Jr. PhD, MS
Division of Diabetes Translation
National Center for Chronic Disease
    Prevention and Health Promotion
Centers for Disease Control and Prevention
Atlanta, GA

Joe Jacobs, MD, MPH
Vermont Health Department

Judith H. LaRosa, PhD, RN, FAAN
Department of Preventive Medicine and
    Community Health
SUNY Downstate Medical Center
Brooklyn, NY

Vickie M. Mays, PhD, MSPH
University of California, Los Angeles
Los Angeles, CA

Deborah Parra-Medina, MPH, PhD
University of South Carolina
Norman J. Arnold School of Public Health
Department of Health Promotion and
    Education and Women's Studies Program
Columbia, SC

Ninez A. Ponce, PhD, MPP
University of California, Los Angeles
School of Public Health
Los Angeles, CA

Neil R. Powe, MD, MPH, MBA
Welch Center for Prevention Epidemiology,
    and Clinical Research
Johns Hopkins Medical Institutions
Department of Epidemiology
Johns Hopkins Bloomberg School of Public
    Health
Baltimore, MD

Mercedes Rubio, PhD
University of Michigan
Department of Sociology
Ann Arbor, MI

Richard R. Sharp, PhD
National Institute of Environmental Health
    Sciences
National Institutes of Health
Research Triangle Park, NC

Douglas H. Ubelaker, PhD
Department of Anthropology
NMNH, MRC 112
Smithsonian Institution
Washington, DC

J. DeWitt Webster, MPH, CHES
The Pennsylvania State University
Department of Biobehavioral Health
College of Health and Human Development
University Park, PA

Joel S. Weissman, PhD
Institute for Health Policy
Massachusetts General Hospital
Boston, MA

Alan L. Wells, MPH
Clinical Ethics Fellow
University of Texas—Houston
School of Public Health
Houston, TX

David R. Williams, PhD
University of Michigan
Department of Sociology
Ann Arbor, MI

PREFACE

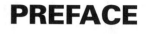

*I*n 1993, the National Institutes of Health created and implemented controversial guidelines mandating the inclusion of women and ethnic minorities in federally funded studies. Despite this legislation, the rate of participation in health studies by people of color has not achieved racial equivalence. More recent support for the inclusion of ethnic minority groups is evidenced by the Strategic Plans for Reducing the Health Disparities developed by each institute at the National Institutes of Health. The consequences of continued underrepresentation may have grave implications for continued unequal emphasis on health and an inequitable base of knowledge regarding treatment modalities.

Historically, ethnic minority participation in health studies has been disproportionately low relative to members of the majority population. This situation has created not only a health disparity, but also a participation disparity in clinical trials. Reasons for the lack of participation have been articulated in an extensive body of scientific literature as well as in the lay print media; despite substantial coverage, the debate has centered on individual factors, focusing on either the practitioner or potential participant, or on systemic factors such as organizational barriers to participation. Broad sociologic factors that potentially have a more indirect, but significant, impact on participation of ethnic minorities in health studies have been largely overlooked. The purpose of this book, therefore, is to examine the lack of minority participation in health studies from social, historical, and scientific perspectives. Toward this end, several interrelated factors that contribute to minimal participation in health studies are considered: past atrocities in medical experimentation, cultural differences in health beliefs and practices, imbalance of power, communication challenges, and issues related to health system organization. A clearer understanding of the reasons underlying the problem of minority participation may bring us closer to achieving the national public health goal of reducing health disparities between the majority and minority populations.

Race and Research: Perspectives on Minority Participation in Health Studies is a teaching text and resource guide for students, health professionals, public health researchers, and the general public that extends the discussion of environmental factors that influence ethnic minority participation in health studies. This book is not meant to be a definitive discussion on all aspects of minority participation in health studies, or a discussion of participation issues regarding minority populations outside the United States. Further, this book is not meant to provide specific strategies on how to successfully recruit minority participants.

This book is divided into three main sections: I) The Meaning of Race, Culture, and Ethnicity in Research; II) Health Studies and Ethnic Minority Populations; and III) The Impact of Revolutionary Changes in Medicine and Health Care on Minority Participation in Health Studies.

Section I includes three chapters. The first, written from an anthropological perspective, addresses the fundamental meaning of the term "race" in science and the common confusion between the social definition of race and accepted scientific variations in human biology. Chapter 2 extends this discussion to question the validity of classifying people in health research as well as the effect of this imprecise measurement approach in a scientific context. Chapter 3 presents the ethical issues in research and a review of well-known and infamous clinical trial abuses in various ethnic populations. Further, this chapter will explore why ethnic minority populations are often "prey" for these studies.

Section II of the book begins with Chapter 4; this chapter presents an overview of the clinical trial, the most rigorous type of study design. Chapter 4 also addresses common concerns of ethnic minority groups regarding the conditions and methods used by these types of studies (such as randomization) and general concerns about human experimentation. Chapter 5 outlines reasons why knowledge about health conditions and the practices of various populations are important to our understanding of diseases and conditions that affect certain groups. The chapter will further describe issues with sampling methods employed in large cohort studies by federal agencies and the degree to which variation between and among ethnic groups may be studied with these data.

Chapter 6 presents the differences in cultural, social, and ethnic variation of health behavior and how the use of traditional theories in behavioral studies may serve to alienate participants because of a lack of inclusion of culturally relevant paradigms. Chapter 7 discusses the ethical issues raised regarding privacy and the confidentiality of collecting data at the molecular level. The contribution of genetic evidence regarding racial admixture toward the understanding of differential morbidity and mortality is also considered. Chapter 8 concludes the second section of the book. This section embraces the discussions in the preceding chapters and outlines the meaning of and need for community capacity for the successful conduct of research in minority populations.

Section III examines the impact of broad changes in medicine and health care that have affected the arena in which health studies are conducted and how these changes have potentially effected minority participation. Chapter 9 is a retrospective examination of why the 1993 NIH Revitalization Act was developed and implemented and the subsequent effect of that act on the conduct of research regarding the targeted population groups. Chapter 10 presents an examination of a relatively new phenomenon: the proliferation of for-profit clinical trials and their effect on trials conducted at academic health centers, which traditionally have had access to a large numbers of ethnic minority populations. Chapter 11 furthers this discussion with an overview of the emergence of managed care and its relative impact on the conduct of research at academic health centers. Finally, Chapter 12 examines the growth and rising acceptability of complementary and alternative medicine (CAM); this chapter further introduces CAM as a fundamental aspect of health behavior that may potentially affect patient compliance, patient–provider communication, and participation in health studies.

ACKNOWLEDGMENTS

At the beginning of this book project, we did not imagine how much time or how many people it would take to carry it through to completion. To all those who wrote chapters, offered advice and expertise, assisted with research, took care of administrative work, participated in our marathon phone calls, endured our initial excitement and, later, our angst over the great deal of work and worry that goes into editing a volume, we thank you from the bottom of our hearts.

We offer special thanks to Dr. Valerie Setlow Wilson, who generously offered her time and experience in the early developmental stages; we felt an incredible synergy working with Val as we determined the organization of the book, the chapter topics, and the authors invited to contribute to the volume. Dr. Wilson helped tremendously with the conceptual work and early details, but equally important were her coaching and reinforcement, which contributed greatly to our confidence to move ahead with the project.

We also offer special thanks to our administrative assistant, Patricia Kirsch Duboue, a perfect picture of efficiency. Patricia stayed with us from beginning to end, always ready to help with whatever needed to be done. To our student assistants, Katie Nevin, MD, MPH, Shirin Madad, MPH, Jaqueline Mosely, MPH, and Gianni Amato, MHA, thank you for wanting to be a part of this project and for your hard work in the libraries and on the Internet.

Much of the work that went into the development of this book was conducted when both editors were colleagues at Tulane University School of Public Health and Tropical Medicine. We would particularly like to thank Drs. Paul Whelton and Judie La Rosa for their encouragement and support.

We extend our special thanks to Joe Jacobs, MD, who generously offered his expertise in the field of complementary and alternative therapies during the composition and refinement of that chapter. Additionally, we extend our sincere appreciation to our reviewers, Drs. Shiriki Kumanyika, Robert Goodman, Stephanie Tortu, and Ann Marie Myers. We thank Dr. Carl Kendall who remained an important source of expert advice, friendship, and encouragement throughout the project. And a wholehearted thank you goes to Dr. Victoria Taylor for her very competent assistance in the "Memphis Office."

We especially thank Ellen Meyer, Director of Publications for the American Public Health Association, and the APHA Publications Board for their endorsement and support of this book. We also thank every author who contributed to this volume; words are not sufficient to express our sincere appreciation for your willingness to join us in this endeavor.

We must also acknowledge the countless scholars of race and minority participation in health studies; we have learned from their work as we researched our topics. Most importantly, we have learned from the minority subjects of health studies whose experiences are chronicled in the literature. For their altruism and willingness to help advance medical science, we wish to formally acknowledge their past, present, and future participation in health research.

Last, but not least, we must thank our spouses, Dr. Derrick Beech and Dr. Alan Goodman. They have lived with us through this project, often enduring our ups and downs, but always ready to offer encouragement and advice.

We sincerely hope this book will make a contribution, however small, toward the design and conduct of health studies that invite and sustain greater minority participation.

Bettina Beech, DrPH, MPH
and Maurine Goodman, MA, MPH

Chapter 1

THE SOCIAL DIMENSION *of* RACE

Mercedes Rubio, PhD,
and David R. Williams, PhD

R ace is a routinely used and widely accepted category that has social, political, psychological, and economic implications. Although many scientists have aban-doned the term as a valid taxonomy for capturing biological variation, the public continues to accept race as a way to understand perceived differences and variations between humans (Muir 1993). For many, "race" explains social and institutional arrangements since it provides an understandable basis for differences in mental abil-ities, aptitudes, and superiority and subordination of groups (Muir 1993). Assumptions about racial groups have profound implications for the way in which societal rewards and resources are distributed. In this chapter we examine race as a socially constructed phenomenon. We begin by providing an overview of how racial categories have been constructed by the census, both within the United States and in other countries. We then examine how the scientific understanding of race has changed over time, and we discuss social dimensions of race as part of the fabric of the American social con-text. An examination of societal dimensions of race in health and health care is also provided. Lastly, we provide guidelines for future research that promote a better understanding of race in health.

History of Measuring Race in the U.S.

The federal government has played a vital role in perpetuating the acceptance of race as a valid construct; over the last two centuries, the Census Bureau has regu-larly defined and redefined racial categories. In 1790, the first census taken in com-pliance with Article 1, Section 2, of the Constitution enumerated free persons, excluding Indians not taxed, and all others (that is, Black slaves) as three-fifths of a

Preparation of this chapter was supported in part by grant T32 MH 16806 from the National Institute of Mental Health.

person (Wright 1966). The Three-Fifths Rule was abandoned by the Thirteenth Amendment and the distinction continued to be made between "civilized Indians" and "Indians not taxed" until 1924 when Congress granted U.S. citizenship to American Indians (Anderson and Feinberg 1995). In each subsequent census, racial category options were expanded and shortened, often reflecting political, economic, and immigration policies of the time (Anderson 1988; Barrera 1979).

The inclusion of particular race categories in the census at certain times versus others has often reflected which immigrant groups were welcomed or unwelcomed on U.S. shores. As large numbers of Chinese migrated to the U.S. in the mid-19th century, Chinese was added as a new racial group in the 1870 Census; a little more than a decade later (1882), the Chinese Exclusion Act barred immigration from China. Similarly, Japanese was added as a new racial category in the 1890 Census to track these new immigrants, and, by 1908, the Gentlemen's Agreement restricted the number of Japanese immigrants.

The assessment of race throughout the 20th century continued to reflect larger social and political realities (Lee 1993). In 1900, the census recognized five racial groups—White, Black, Chinese, Japanese, and Indian. In both the 1910 and 1920 censuses, Mulatto was included as a race category. Census data continued to figure prominently in immigration policy (Barrera 1979). The Quota Law of 1921 established quotas for immigration based on the nationality of immigrants already in the U.S. based on the 1910 Census, and the 1924 Immigration Act set new quotas based on the proportion of various nationalities in the U.S. based on the 1890 Census. The 1930 Census included for the first time Mexican, Filipino, Hindu, and Korean as race options. The estimate of the Mexican-descent population in the 1930 Census coincided with the implementation of the Repatriation Act of 1930, which initiated a federally sponsored program to apprehend and deport Mexicans and Mexican-Americans who could not prove that they were legally in the U.S. (Barrera 1979). Whether intentionally racist or not, immigration policies have helped to reinforce long-standing racial ideology in the U.S.

However, by the 1940 Census, Mexicans were, for the first time, classified as White. The 1950 Census shortened the list of racial categories to include only White, Negro, American Indian, Japanese, Chinese, Filipino, and Other. The 1960 Census recognized eleven racial categories, adding Hawaiian, Part-Hawaiian, Aleut, and Eskimo to the 1950 classifications. Census enumerators were instructed to designate Puerto Ricans, Mexicans, and other persons of Latin descent as White when it was evident, based on observation, that they were definitely not Negro. The 1970 Census allowed respondents to choose which racial category they identified with, but the recognized racial categories were White, Negro or Black, American Indian, Japanese, Chinese, Filipino, Hawaiian, Korean, and Other.

In 1978, the federal government's Office of Management and Budget (OMB) published guidelines for the uniform assessment of race and ethnicity by federal statistical agencies. These guidelines recognized four racial groups, White, Black, American Indian or Alaskan Native, and Asian or Pacific Islander (API), and one ethnic category, Hispanic. The racial classifications for the 1980 and 1990 censuses used these categories. The OMB guidelines are minimal standards, and the census has collect-ed additional detail for some categories. For example, additional subgroups identi-fied in the API category include Chinese, Filipino, Hawaiian, Korean, Vietnamese, Japanese, Asian Indian, Samoan, and Guamanian.

Prior to the 2000 Census, there was considerable debate regarding how race eth-nicity should be conceptualized and measured (Evinger 1995). The OMB faced crit-icism that the official racial and ethnic categories no longer reflected the growing racial and ethnic diversity of the U.S. Some proposed the elimination of any attempt to classify persons by race. Additionally, there was disagreement over the optimal terminology to be used for various racial groups, whether a new multiracial catego-ry should be utilized for persons of mixed racial ancestry, whether new categories should be added for persons from the Middle East or the Cape Verde islands, whether Native Hawaiians should be classified with American Indians instead of with the API category, and whether Hispanic should be a racial or an ethnic category.

In an effort to address the concerns of various interest groups, the Census Bureau collaborated with other federal agencies to collect more information on the public's preferences for the assessment of race and ethnic origin in three major data collec-tion efforts. One of the goals was to test the multiracial and "Hispanic" race cate-gories (Tucker and Kojetin 1996). An important finding from this research was that the size of some racial and ethnic populations varied depending on how the race questions were asked. For example, almost 80% of those surveyed categorized them-selves as White when race and Hispanic origin questions were asked separately com-pared to approximately 76% when Hispanic origin was included as a racial catego-ry. Also, a higher percentage of persons identified themselves as Hispanic when they were asked a separate Hispanic origin question than when there was a combined race and ethnic origin question. Similarly, including a multiracial category resulted in a 25% reduction in the size of the American Indian population.

The distribution within the Latino population also changed depending on how race was assessed. There were differences in the distribution of people of Mexican descent and of Cubans depending on how questions were asked. For example, 60% of Hispanic respondents identified with being Mexican when race and Hispanic ori-gin were asked separately, compared to 67% when race and Hispanic origin were combined. In contrast, there was a decrease in the Cuban percentages; approximately 5% of Latinos identified as Cuban when race and Hispanic origin were assessed sep-arately compared to 2% when the race and Hispanic origin questions were combined (Tucker and Kojetin 1996).

Based on the testing of racial and ethnic origin questions and other political con-siderations, OMB published new guidelines for "Maintaining, Collecting, and Presenting Federal Data on Race and Ethnicity" in the *Federal Register*, October 30, 1997. The most radical change in the new federal standard will allow persons of mixed-racial ancestry to list themselves in as many racial categories as apply. Data on multiracial status have been collected in earlier censuses. The 1890 Census includ-ed the mixed-race categories Mulatto, Quadroon, and Octoroon. These were dropped in 1900 but Mulatto reappeared as a race option in both the 1910 and 1920 Censuses

(Lee 1993). Other changes include the expansion of the racial categories by one, with Native Hawaiian and Other Pacific Islander constituting a new racial category separate from Asian. Hispanic has been retained as an ethnic category, and Hispanic origin will be assessed prior to race in the census. In addition, changes in terminology allow for "Black or African-American" and "Hispanic or Latino" to be utilized. These new guidelines are being utilized by the 2000 Census and will be implemented in all federal data systems by 2003. The federal classification of race and ethnicity reflect past and present political and ideological struggles, and they have important implications for popular conceptualizations of race, how different racial/ethnic groups interact and perceive one another, how resources are distributed, and how health status is measured (Lee 1993).

Race in Canada and the United Kingdom

Like the U.S., both Canada and the United Kingdom are dealing with challenges with regard to the assessment of race and ethnicity. Canada, like the U.S., has changed its racial/ethnic categories depending on social and political circumstances. As the population increased in diversity, the census racial/ethnic categories began to reflect it, albeit at a much slower pace. The 1871 Canadian Census used English, Irish, Scotch, African, Indian, German, and French as racial and ethnic origin categories (Kralt 1980). In the 1891 Census no racial questions were asked. However, the 1901 Census expanded the race options to include White (based on father's race), Japanese, Chinese, Negro, Indians (enumerated based on tribal affiliation), and individuals of mixed heritage (Kralt 1980). The 1971 Census measured ethnicity, based on paternal ancestry for all residents of Canada, except for Native Indians. White respondents were provided with options such as English, French, Scottish, Polish, German, Jewish, etc. However, only single ethnic origin responses were accepted (Kralt 1980; Pryor, Goldmann, and Royce 1991). By 1981, multiple racial/ethnic responses were tolerated; by 1986, they were encouraged. In 1986, changes were made to the ethnic origin question. Prior to 1986 respondents were asked the ethnic or cultural group to which they belonged "on first coming to this continent." In 1986 the phrase "on first coming to this continent" was dropped, and "Black" was reintroduced as a category (Pryor, Goldmann, and Royce 1991).

Like the U.S., the types of questions and categories used to assess race in the U.K. is a pragmatic compromise from among a variety of competing ideological pressures and interest groups. The 1991 U.K. Census was the first to assess race. Prior censuses collected data only on country of birth. The 1991 U.K. Census was surrounded with similar debates as those in the U.S. in the mid 1990s (Ballard 1997). One of the objectives of the 1991 U.K. Census was not so much to explore the ethnic diversity of the country, but to determine what percentage was non-European.

As such, the 1991 U.K. Census asked the population to identify as White (without any further specification of ethnic affiliation) or with one of six pre-assigned ethno-national categories: Black Caribbean, Black African, Indian, Pakistani, Bangladeshi, or Chinese. An additional 28 categories were developed in the census based on write-in responses to the "Black—Other" and the residual "Any Other

Ethnic Group" categories. Many tabulations of census data used the seven preset codes and three additional categories: Black Others, Other Asian, and Other. Ballard (1997) has criticized the approach taken by the U.K., arguing that:

> while the census has certainly generated, as was intended, a convenient means of identifying the newer and more visible minorities, it has by no means cracked the broader issues. Indeed, given the built-in conceptual deficiencies in the whole process, which both reflect and reinforce the hegemonic impact of racist and anglocentric assumptions, it is hard to be confident that the new initiative will lead to a more accurate charting of the wider terrain. On the contrary, what we may be well witnessing is the construction and institutionalization of a conceptual vision which actually reinforces all the most misleading aspects of popular assumptions about racial and ethnic diversity (p. 193).

The assessment of racial and ethnic status in the U.S., Canada, and the U.K. tends to focus on classifying readily visible nondominant population groups, while the White category goes uncontested. This method of categorizing people can encourage the division of groups based on skin color, reinforce racial stereotypes, and obscure the heterogeneity that exists within the White label.

What Is Race? A Historical Perspective

Francois Bernier, a French physician, introduced the term race into science in 1684. Race, for him, captured differences in skin color, hair, and facial features, and value judgments were made based on these differences (Muir 1993). At about the same time when Bernier wrote about the "four or five species or races of men," many European powers were expanding their colonial empires, and the perceived differences between the "races of men" reinforced European notions that their social arrangements and culture (religion, moral codes, and sexual practices) were superior to those of groups of darker color. These notions of superiority provided, at least in part, the justification for the exploitation of groups regarded as inferior (Muir 1993; Jordan 1968).

When the Europeans arrived in America, they saw the indigenous people as a labor source. However, since many Native American tribes were victims of genocide by brutality and disease, White immigrants filled the labor shortage for a time by entering into a contractual agreement to serve as indentured servants for a specified number of years (Jordan 1968). As the colonies developed, indentured servitude did not meet the labor demands, and the Europeans turned to Africa as a source of labor, partly because of a perceived need for some kind of cheap, bound, labor and partly because Africa and Africans were devalued (Jordan 1968). The U.S. created a system where slave status was associated with dark skin color—first with indigenous people and then with Blacks—and where freedom was associated with White skin. This arrangement based on skin color was advantageous to the slave owners, who encouraged the development of stereotypes based on color. Therefore, it can be argued that from the inception of the United States, a racial ideology has existed with Whites at the top, Blacks at the bottom, and other groups in between. This racial ideology was, and continues to be, a system of beliefs where notions of superiority and inferiority are ascribed based on readily evident external characteristics.

Kreiger (1987) shows that 19th century medical research was used to reinforce the inferiority of Blacks and provide a "scientific" justification for slavery and economic exploitation. One research team falsified insanity rates from the 1840 census to show that rates of mental illness increased among Blacks as they lived further north. This was interpreted as strong evidence that Blacks were biologically suited for slavery such that freedom actually made Blacks crazy! Other specific psychiatric disorders of Blacks identified by 19th century medical researchers included "drapeto-mania," a virulent form of mental illness that led to a desire to escape from slavery, and "dysesthesia Ethiopia," a medical condition, easily identifiable by slave masters, that led to attempts to avoid work or to sleep during the day.

After the end of slavery in 1863, those who wanted to maintain control over their former slaves found new ways of doing so. To some extent they relied on science (biology, anthropology, medicine) to provide a "biological" justification for the subjugation of Blacks and other people of color. Common stereotypes from slavery are reflected in "images portraying Blacks as childlike and irresponsible, inefficient, lazy, ridiculous in speech, pleasure seeking, and happy" (Muir 1993, p. 343). Biological justifications coupled with stereotypes based on color were often used as the basis for assumptions about the culture, morality, behavior, and the intelligence of darker skinned peoples. Links between cultural and social status through perceived biological differences were the basis for "Jim Crow" and "separate but equal" laws defined by the color line. Thus, one's race became a central determinant of access to societal resources and rewards.

The scientific understanding of race has changed over time. It is important to note that the concept of race predates modern theories of genetics and well executed genetic studies. Instead, the term reflects a sociopolitical understanding of human diversity, rather than a biological one. The re-evaluation of race as a biological category (representing distinctive genetic make-up) is based on two grounds. First, there is no firm scientific basis or method for racial taxonomy (Montagu 1964), that is, there are no scientific criteria that can be uniformly used to classify persons into mutually exclusive racial categories. Second, phenotypic characteristics used to define race are not strongly associated with genotypic variations (Muir 1993). For example, phenotypic characteristics (i.e., facial features, hair and skin color, or any other external physical characteristic) are not related to biochemical or other genetic characteristic (Littlefield, Lieberman, and Reynolds 1982; Gould 1977). Differences that may exist between groups tend to reflect environmental adaptation, or genetic exchanges between groups, rather than static genetic differences. Lewontin (1991, p. 37) explains that "about 85 percent of all identified human genetic variation is between any two individuals from the same ethnic group. Another 8% of all the variations is between ethnic groups within a race and only 7% of all human genetic variations lies on the average between major races" (p. 37). As Kreiger and Bassett (1986) have cogently argued, the fact that we know what race we belong to tells us more about our society than about our genetic makeup.

LaVeist (1994) and Williams (1997) have shown that a change in the scientific understanding of race is readily evident by examining the definition of race in scientific dictionaries. Social science dictionaries published in the 1960s or earlier tend to uniformly view race as a valid way of capturing biological and physical variations in human population groups. In contrast, more recent definitions of race question the traditional assumptions of biological homogeneity and propose that race is an unscientific term (e.g., Jary and Jary 1991). Other definitions indicate that race is socially constructed since available scientific evidence does not support the earlier biological view of race (e.g., Seymour-Smith 1986).

A study of physical anthropology textbooks published between 1932 and 1979 revealed that, while early textbooks viewed race as a valid taxonomy for describing human variation, later textbooks increasingly took the position that races do not exist (Littlefield, Lieberman, and Reynolds 1982). Physical anthropologists still agree that there is considerable biological variation in human populations. However, these biological traits are distributed across our "racial" boundaries, and cline is the preferred term to capture human genetic variations. Intriguingly, the scientific data discrediting race as a useful way to capture genetic homogeneity were available long before the race concept was abandoned (Montagu 1964). Goodman (1997) argues, for example, that "race should have been discarded at the turn of the century, when the American anthropologist Franz Boas showed that race, language, and culture do not go hand-in-hand, as raciologists had contended" (p. 21). It was changes in the discipline of physical anthropology (the number of departments, the social class background of the faculty, and the larger cultural context) that led to changes in the discipline (Littlefield, Lieberman, and Reynolds 1982).

Williams (1997) shows that although recent definitions of race in the social sciences have moved away from a biological view, dictionaries in medicine and public health have clung to the scientifically discredited biological position; for example, the third edition of the *Dictionary of Epidemiology* (Last 1995) defines race as "persons who are relatively homogeneous with respect to biological inheritance." Why do some scientific disciplines resist accepting well-established scientific evidence on the nature of race? Some ways of viewing race are more consistent with certain world views and more consonant with the status quo. Duster (1984) emphasizes that conceptions of race that emphasize biological differences are least threatening to the existing societal arrangements.

Thus, although not necessarily intended by individual researchers, a focus on biological sources for racial variations in health can play an important ideological role in the larger society. If racial ethnic differences in health result from innate biological differences, then social institutions and policies that may play a crucial role in determining health status are absolved from responsibility and can remain intact (Lewontin 1991). When problems of health and disease are located within the individual without any attention to the larger social context, the individual becomes the problem and the focus for intervention while attention is diverted from the social forces that can also contribute to disease. Thus, a biological perspective alone is inadequate to explain the unequal distribution of health across various social statuses, including race (Lewontin 1991). In fact, Cooper (1984) has demonstrated that diseases that have a strong genetic component explain less than one percent of the total excess health burden of the Black population compared to the White population in the United States.

More generally, Duster (1984) emphasizes that science is not value-free and that preconceived opinions, cultural norms, and political agendas often shape scientific research by determining what questions are asked and what questions are neglected. He cites several historical instances where social influences played a large role in scientific agendas. The use of the IQ test is one example. At the turn of the 20th century, as the stream of European immigrants changed from persons of English, Scandinavian, and German background to those of Italian, Jewish, Polish, and Russian backgrounds, IQ tests were administered to the new immigrants and lower scores for Southern European immigrants were regarded as evidence of their genetic inferiority and feeble mindedness (Duster 1984; Lieberson 1980). Accordingly, in the 1920s U.S. immigration policy was changed in an effort to reduce the number of Southern European immigrants to the United States.

Later in the century, as a large number of Blacks migrated from the south to the north, Blacks became an increasing economic threat to working-class Whites (Lieberson 1980). IQ tests revealed that Blacks had lower scores than Whites. Duster (1984) notes that, at the same time, IQ tests also revealed that Gentiles tended to score more poorly than Jews. The trajectory of these two findings was very different. In the case of the Jewish/Gentile disparity, the differences were immediately dismissed as due to cultural factors and not widely publicized. In contrast, the Black/White difference was widely cited as evidence of the genetic inferiority of Blacks. New research agendas were developed and funded in this area of inquiry. Jensen (1969) and others argued that because the IQ differences were due to heredity, government-sponsored compensatory education programs intended to assist Blacks were a waste of time. The key point emphasized by Duster (1984) is that the social and political context explains the nature, direction, and trajectory of research on Black/White differences in intelligence.

Goodman (1997) cites research by Giles and Elliot (1962) as an example from forensic science that indicates the extent to which a particular body of scientific information consistent with societal understandings of race continues to be widely used and cited even when discredited by more recent scientific inquiry. These researchers measured the skulls of Black and White males that died in Missouri and Ohio at the turn of the century, and the skulls of Native Americans from a prehistoric site in Kentucky. The researchers developed a mathematical equation based on eight measurements that could be used to identify the race of an individual based on skull size once its gender was known, and that about 80 to 90 percent of the time their racial classification would match the one assigned at the time of death. These measurements have been widely used by forensic scientists and practitioners to identify racial status in forensic investigations. However, Goodman (1997) indicates that when Giles' and Elliott's formula was retested outside Missouri, Ohio, and Kentucky it was found to be less accurate than random assignment of race to various skulls. Given the degree of variation within racial and ethnic populations, many persons belonging to a given racial category diverge from the "ideal type."

The Tuskegee syphilis study also illustrates how normative beliefs about race can lead to hypotheses and the initiation of a research project that scientists would normally rule out (Brandt 1978). This study was initiated in 1932 to identify the health consequences of leaving syphilis untreated in Black males. Dr. Joseph Earl Moore, a key member of the Tuskegee research study team, published papers in which he advocated treatment of syphilis in its latent stages and the absence of any need for a study of untreated syphilis (Brandt 1978). His participation in the Tuskegee study was possible only because of the prevailing conceptualization of race at the time. Conventional scientific wisdom regarded Blacks as morally inferior to Whites with exaggerated libido, widespread sexual promiscuity, and a reluctance to seek treatment for latent syphilis because it was asymptomatic. Most importantly, though, the conventional scientific view was that Blacks and Whites were so different biologically that any disease, including syphilis, would be a different clinical entity in Blacks compared to Whites. Accordingly, the findings from the earlier Oslo study of untreated syphilis, which was the source of Dr. Moore's assertions, could not be generalized to Blacks because they came from a population of Whites. Accordingly, this long-term follow-up study of untreated syphilis in Black males used multiple strategies of deception to recruit subjects and ensure compliance. Moreover, it not only withheld treatment from participants but went to elaborate lengths to ensure that they did not otherwise receive treatment.

Social Dimensions of Race in Contemporary America

More than 50 years ago, Cox (1948) emphasized that stigmatizing a socially marginalized racial group as inferior was a critical step in justifying the exploitation of that group or its resources. Negative attitudes by Whites toward people of color have been longstanding in the U.S. These attitudes and the ideology of inferiority that has undergirded them have played a role in creating social policies that have determined the access of non-Whites to societal goods and ultimately to health status and health care.

Data on racial attitudes over time provide compelling evidence of major changes in racial prejudice in the U.S. (Shuman et al. 1997). These data reveal that an overwhelming majority of Whites now endorse egalitarian values and are, in principle, opposed to segregation in residential and educational contexts and discrimination in multiple domains of society. Two examples will suffice. In 1963, 60% of Whites agreed that they had the right to keep Blacks out of their neighborhoods if they wanted to, but only 13% of Whites supported that view by 1996. Similarly, in 1944, more than half of all Whites (55%) indicated that White people should have the first chance at any kind of job. By 1972, only 3% of Whites agreed with that view, with 97% indicating that Blacks should have as good a chance as White people to get any kind of job. This positive change in the attitudes of Whites toward Blacks concerning equal treatment in job opportunities, housing, and education is impressive.

Moreover, these positive shifts in public sentiments were given the force of law through various civil rights statutes. The Civil Rights Act of 1964 (which outlawed racial discrimination in employment), the Voting Rights Act of 1965, and the Civil

Rights Act of 1968 (which outlawed racial discrimination in the sale or rental of housing) are examples of laws that attempted to establish a color-blind society. Some believe that the combination of the legal system and the court of public opinion would eliminate widespread racism in the U.S. However, closer analysis reveals that the picture is more complex and that reports of the death of discrimination may be grossly exaggerated. First, although Whites support the principle of equality in general, they are less supportive of the policies that would implement them. For example, Shuman et al. (1997) show that in 1964, 38% of Whites indicated that the government in Washington should see to it that Black people got fair treatment in jobs, and 13% indicated that they lacked enough interest in the question to favor one side over another. By 1996, the percentage of Whites supporting federal intervention to ensure fair treatment in jobs declined to 28%, while the percentage expressing no interest in the question increased to 36%. Hence, Shuman et al. (1997) argue that this gap between principles and implementation is at the heart of the enduring inequality between the two populations.

Second, other data reveal that Whites continue to hold very negative views of Blacks and other minorities. Table 1 presents stereotype data from the 1990 General Social Survey, a highly respected national social indicators study (Davis and Smith 1990). The first column indicates that 44% of Whites perceive Blacks as lazy, and over 50% perceive that Blacks prefer to live on welfare and are prone to violence. Further, 20% or less of Whites endorsed positive stereotypes about African-Americans

Table 1. White Americans' Stereotypes
Percent Agreeing With Most Group Members...

	Blacks	Whites	Hispanics	Asians
Are Unintelligent				
Unintelligent	28.8	6.1	29.1	13.2
Neither	45.0	33.3	42.6	38.0
Intelligent	20.0	55.4	18.4	37.3
DK/NA	6.2	5.2	9.8	11.5
Are Lazy				
Lazy	44.3	4.9	33.5	15.0
Neither	34.0	36.4	33.7	27.7
Hardworking	16.8	54.5	23.9	47.2
DK/NA	4.9	4.2	9.0	10.1
Prefer Welfare				
Prefer welfare	56.1	3.7	41.6	16.3
Neither	26.5	21.5	30.5	31.6
Prefer self support	12.7	70.5	18.3	40.6
DK/NA	4.7	4.3	9.7	11.5
Are Prone to Violence				
Violence prone	50.5	15.7	38.3	17.2
Neither	28.3	42.3	34.0	41.1
Not violence prone	15.2	36.6	17.8	29.6
DK/NA	5.9	5.5	9.8	12.1

Source: Davis and Smith 1990.
DK/NA: Don't know or no answer.

(only 20% believed that Blacks were intelligent, 17% that they were hardworking, 13 percent that Blacks were self-supporting, and 15% that Blacks were not prone to violence). In addition, a substantial percentage of White respondents opted for the socially acceptable "neither" response category.

These negative perceptions are especially striking when compared to how Whites view themselves. Comparatively, Whites believe that only 4% of Whites prefer to live on welfare, 16% are prone to violence, 6% are unintelligent, and 5% are lazy. Moreover, Whites viewed Blacks, Hispanics, and Asians more negatively than themselves, with Blacks being viewed more negatively than all other groups, and Hispanics twice as negatively as Asians. These data reveal that perceptions of inferiority about people of color continue to persist.

Such high levels of negative stereotypes are likely to have profound implications in situations ranging from personal day-to-day interactions to public policy. Research on stereotypes indicates that the endorsement of negative racial stereotypes leads to discrimination against minority groups (Devine 1995; Hilton and von Hippel 1996). Biases based on racial stereotypes occur automatically and without conscious awareness (Devine 1989; Hilton and von Hippel 1996). That is, the activation of these stereotypes and the discrimination linked to them is an automatic process with individuals spontaneously becoming aware of relevant stereotypes after encountering someone to whom the stereotypes are applicable. This means that much contemporary discriminatory behavior is unconscious—it occurs through behaviors that the perpetrator does not subjectively experience as intentional. Thus, the high level of negative stereotyping suggests that racial discrimination is a widespread societal problem and not just the aberrant behavior of a few "bad apples."

Institutional Discrimination and Access to Societal Rewards

This insight is critical to understanding the often paradoxical contemporary data on race in the U.S. An integral part of maintaining the social order and White structural privilege is racism—an organized system, rooted in an ideology of inferiority that categorizes, ranks, and differentially allocates societal resources to various population groups (Bonilla-Silva 1996); it may or may not be accompanied by prejudice at the individual level. Racism appears to have changed over time from blatant "Jim Crow racism" that emphasized biological differences between the races to a more subtle "laissez-faire racism" (Bobo, Kluegel, and Smith 1997). This new racism focuses on the perceived cultural inferiority of minorities (lack of the traditional values, motivation, and behavioral strategies required for success), but it occurs within the context of a strong endorsement of equality without a corresponding commitment to achieve it.

Although racial attitudes have changed, many of the institutional structures (such as residential segregation) that ensured that nondominant racial groups had differential access to power and desirable resources remain intact. Moreover, the persistence of racial stereotypes in the U.S. provides a critical reservoir for the maintenance of racial discrimination, and research reveals that racial stereotypes have real-life consequences for minority groups' access to societal resources. Based on negative stereotypes of African-Americans, the majority of Whites express a strong preference for living in racially segregated neighborhoods (Williams et al. 1999; Bobo and Zubrinsky 1996), and Blacks in search of housing are steered toward neighborhoods having a greater number of minorities, lower home values, and lower median income (Fix and Struyk 1993). A review of the research on housing discrimination in the U.S. concluded that, "On any given encounter between a Black home-seeker and a realtor, the odds are at least 60 percent that something will happen to limit that Black renter or buyer's access to housing units that are available to Whites" (Massey, Gross, and Shibuya 1994, p. 443).

Studies of White employers reveal that racial stereotypes are used to deny employment opportunities to Black applicants (Kirschenman and Neckerman 1991; Neckerman and Kirschenman 1991). In addition, both U.S.–based and foreign companies explicitly use the racial composition of labor markets in deciding where to locate new plants (Cole and Deskins 1988). Other evidence suggests that such institutional discrimination has dire consequences for Blacks' access to employment. For example, a *Wall Street Journal* analysis of the employment records of over 35,000 U.S. companies found that African-Americans had a net job loss of 59,000 jobs during the 1990–91 economic downturn, compared to net gains of 71,100 for Whites, 55,100 for Asians, and 60,000 for Latinos (Sharpe 1993). These job losses reflected the relocation of employment facilities to areas of lower African-American concentration. Audit studies of employment discrimination also document racial differences in application submissions, in obtaining interviews, and in being offered jobs. In these studies, when trained Black and White job applicants with identical qualifications applied for jobs, discrimination favored the White over the Black applicants in one out of five audits (Fix and Struyk 1993).

Race still matters a lot in the U.S. Large racial differences exist in education, housing, health, criminal justice, labor force participation, retirement, pensions, and asset accumulation (Jaynes and Williams 1989; Smelser, Wilson, and Mitchell in press). More disturbing, three decades after the passage of civil rights legislation little advancement has been made in narrowing the racial gap in terms of income, housing, educational quality, and unemployment. The degree of residential racial segregation in 1990 was virtually identical to what it was when Congress passed the Fair Housing Act in 1968 (Massey 1996). Similarly, the unemployment rate for Blacks has been consistently about twice that of Whites from 1950 to the present (*Economic Report of the President* 1998). There has also been remarkable stability over time in the racial inequality in income. For example, the median income of African-Americans was 59 cents for every dollar earned by Whites in 1996—identical to what it was in 1978 (*Economic Report of the President* 1998).

There is also growing recognition that data on income understate racial differences in economic status. Income only captures the flow of economic resources into the household, but does not address the economic reserves of the household. Racial differences in wealth are larger than those for income. For example, White households have a median net worth that is 10 times that of African-American households, and 9 times that of Hispanic households (Eller 1994) these differences persist at all levels of income. Whites in the lowest quintile of income have a median net worth of $10,257 compared to $1 for comparable Blacks and $645 for Hispanics. Similarly, Oliver and Shapiro (1995) found that White households headed by a college graduate had an average net worth of $75,000 compared to $20,000 for a similar Black household (controlling for number of earners in the household, age of head of household, and marital status). Much of the wealth of American families exists in the form of home equity, and the racial difference is thus linked to housing policies and institutional discrimination experienced in the past (Oliver and Shapiro 1995).

More generally, the evidence indicates that socioeconomic status (SES) indicators, whether at the level of the community, the household, or the individual, are not equivalent across racial groups. There is not one city among the 171 largest cities in the United States where Whites live under equivalent conditions to Blacks in terms of rates of poverty and single-parent households (Sampson and Wilson 1995). In many urban areas, the concentration of poverty linked to residential segregation, combined with high rates of male joblessness and residential instability, leads to few opportunities for marriage, high rates of family disruption, and high rates of violent crime. Sampson and Wilson (1995, p. 41) concluded that, "the worst urban context in which Whites reside is considerably better than the average context of Black communities."

Measures of education are not equivalent across race. National data reveal that at every level of education Blacks and Hispanics have lower levels of income than Whites (U.S. Census Bureau 1997). The purchasing power of a given level of income also varies across race. Blacks have higher costs for goods and services than Whites due to higher prices on average for a broad range of services in the central city areas where Blacks live than in suburban areas where most Whites reside (Williams and Collins 1995). There are also large racial differences in economic hardship. National data reveal that even after adjustment for a broad range of economic factors (income, education, transfer payments, home ownership, employment status, disability, and health insurance) and demographic factors (age, gender, marital status, the presence of children, and residential mobility), African-Americans were more likely than Whites to experience the following hardships: unable to meet essential expenses, unable to pay for rent or mortgage, unable to pay full utility bill, had utilities shut off, had telephone service shut off, and evicted from apartment or home (Bauman 1998).

Societal Dimensions of Race in Contemporary Health Care

Health Status of People of Color

Race continues to be a strong predictor of variations in health in the United States. Table 2 illustrates the racial differences in health by presenting death rates for Whites and minority/White ratios for the leading causes of death in 1997. The table shows that Blacks have a death rate from all causes that is 1.5 times higher than that of Whites. Of the 11 specific causes of death in Table 2, the death rates for African-Americans are higher than those of Whites for 9 of the 11 causes of death; pulmonary

Table 2. Age-Adjusted Death Rates for Whites for Leading Causes of Death in the United States for Minority/White Ratios, 1999

Causes	Whites non-Hispanics	White, Non-Hispanic/Minority Ratios			
		Black/ White Ratio	Amer. Indian/ White Ratio	API*/ White Ratio	Hispanic/ White Ratio
All	860.7	1.33	0.83	0.60	0.70
Diseases of the heart	263.3	1.28	0.65	0.59	0.67
Cancer	199.8	1.27	0.63	0.63	0.61
Cerebrovascular diseases	194.5	0.42	0.20	0.27	0.21
Chronic lower respiratory diseases	47.5	0.71	0.64	0.40	0.42
Injuries and accidents	35.5	1.15	1.72	0.50	0.88
Diabetes	22.8	2.20	2.21	0.81	1.47
Influenza and pneumonia	23.4	1.09	0.94	0.67	0.67
Suicide	11.5	0.50	1.03	0.56	0.53
Chronic liver disease and cirrhosis	9.7	1.05	2.91	0.39	1.59
Homicide	3.8	5.42	2.76	0.84	2.21
HIV/AIDS	2.9	8.31	1.07	0.28	2.48

Source: National Center for Health Statistics, 2001, pp.167–168.
* API = Asian/Pacific Islander.

disease and suicide are the two exceptions. Higher death rates of Blacks compared to Whites range from 1.2 times higher for injuries and accidents to 8 times higher for homicide and legal intervention and 9.6 times higher for HIV/AIDS. This clear pattern of elevated death rates across a broad range of major health outcomes also suggests that no single gene or biological factor is implicated. Moreover, whatever the major underlying factors for the excess deaths of the African-American population are, they appear to remain potent over time. Our earliest mortality data reveal that Blacks in the United States have always had higher death rates than Whites, and some evidence suggest that the overall Black/White differences are widening with time. For example, Williams (1999a) recently showed that the Black/White ratios for death rates for heart diseases, cancer, diabetes, and cirrhosis of the liver were larger in 1995 than they were in 1950. This reflected a more rapid decline of death rates for some causes for Whites than Blacks (for example, heart disease) and relatively stable death rates for Whites for other causes compared with increasing death rates for Blacks (for example, cancer).

Native Americans have an overall death rate that is virtually identical to that of Whites. However, when we look at specific causes of death, some are considerably lower for the Native American population compared to the White population (for example, stroke, cancer, and pulmonary disease) while others are considerably higher. Compared to Whites, Native Americans are about 3 times more likely to die of heart disease, liver disease, and homicide and legal intervention, 2.7 times more likely to die of diabetes, and 2 times more likely to die from injuries and accidents. The Asian or Pacific Islander population and the Hispanic population have an overall death rate that is lower than that of the White population. For virtually all causes of death, death rates for Asians are lower than those of Whites. The only exceptions are homicide and legal intervention, which is 1.2 times higher for Asians than the White population, and stroke, where both racial groups have equivalent rates. The Latino population, in contrast, has lower death rates for the leading causes of death (heart disease, cancer, and stroke) than the White population. At the same time, compared to the White population, Latinos have death rates that are 1.8 times higher for liver disease, 1.7 times higher for diabetes, and 3.2 times higher for HIV/AIDS and homicide.

Immigration plays an important role in the lower mortality rates for the Asian and Pacific Islander population and the Latino population. High proportions of both of these groups are immigrants to the United States, and immigrants of all racial and ethnic groups tend to have better health than their native-born counterparts, even when these immigrants are lower in socioeconomic status (Singh and Yu 1996; Hummer et al. 1999). However, with increasing length of stay, the health status of immigrants deteriorates as they often abandon traditional behaviors and values for U.S. mainstream culture (Vega and Amaro 1994).

Racial and ethnic populations are characterized by considerable heterogeneity, and focusing on overall rates for groups often obscures important variability. Table 3 illustrates some of this heterogeneity for infant mortality rates. It presents infant mortality rates for the major racial/ethnic populations in the United States and the minority White ratios. Importantly, it shows multiple subgroups for both the Asian and Pacific Islander and the Hispanic origin categories. The data reveal that compared to non-Hispanic Whites, infant mortality among Black infants is 2.4 times higher, and 1.7 times higher in Native American infants. The Asian or Pacific Islander population has an infant mortality rate that is lower than that of the White population, and the overall Hispanic origin rate is slightly higher than that of the White

Table 3. Infant Mortality Rates According to Race: United States 1996–1998

Race of Mother and Hispanic Origin of Mother	Rates*	White/Non-White Ratio
White, Non-Hispanic	6.0	
Black, Non-Hispanic	13.9	2.32
American Indian or Alaskan Native	9.3	1.55
Asian or Pacific Islander	5.2	0.87
Chinese	3.4	0.57
Japanese	4.3	0.72
Filipino	5.9	0.98
Hawaiian and part Hawaiian	8.2	1.37
Other Asian or Pacific Islander	5.5	0.92
Hispanic Origin	5.9	0.98
Mexican	5.8	0.97
Puerto Rican	8.1	1.35
Cuban	4.7	0.78
Central and South American	5.2	0.87
Other and unknown Hispanic	6.8	1.13

* Infant Deaths per 1,000 live births.
Source: National Center for Health Statistics, 2001, p. 153.

population. Some subgroups within the Asian category, such as Chinese and Japanese, have rates that are considerably lower than that of even the overall Asian category.

However, native Hawaiians have an overall rate that is higher than the Asian and White populations, and Mexicans, Cubans, and Central and South Americans have an infant mortality rate that is lower than that of the overall Hispanic origin population and the White population. In contrast, Puerto Ricans and the Other Hispanic category have rates that are higher than the overall Hispanic origin group, as well as the White population.

The health status of a people is shaped by their social stratification, and thus their life circumstances (Engels 1993 [1884]; Turner, Wheaton, and Lloyd, 1995). Much of the disparity that exists between Whites and non-Whites reflects the life circumstances and social policies that have historically limited the opportunities of disenfranchised groups. Differences in health outcome as an effect of social position and race/ethnicity are not new or unique to the U.S. A robust inverse relationship exists between socioeconomic status and health outcomes in both industrialized and developing countries (Antonovsky 1967; Bunker, Gomby, and Kehrer 1989; Williams 1990; Adler et al. 1993; Marmot et al. 1991). Overall, better health outcomes are associated with higher levels of socioeconomic status.

A prominent hypothesis, in the health literature, is that social class standing accounts for racial variations in health, and this is largely due to SES being a correlate of race. Research has shown that Black/White health differentials are always substantially reduced and sometimes eliminated when social class is adjusted for (Williams and Collins 1995; Lillie-Blanton et al. 1996). Yet, even when indicators of SES such as education or income are statistically controlled, Blacks tend to have poorer health status than Whites (Williams 1999b; Navarro 1991). As noted earlier, all indicators of SES are not equivalent across racial groups, and income understates the true magnitude of racial differences in economic resources. In addition, focusing only on current SES does not address the dynamic nature of SES effects over the life course and the potential role that economic deprivation in early life can play in determining adult health status (Williams and Collins 1995). In addition, a growing body of research suggests that racism can also impact the health of minority populations (Krieger 1999; Williams 1999). Racism can affect health indirectly through SES by reducing employment and educational opportunities. It can also affect health and death directly through the stress of personal experiences of discrimination, via the negative consequences of residence in poor neighborhoods, and through racial bias in medical care.

Access to and Quality of Health Care

Two contributing factors to the higher death rates among non-Whites are access to and quality of health care. Economic factors are commonly cited barriers to health care (Estrada, Trevino, and Ray 1990). Without a doubt, there is a link between employment status and health coverage. High levels of unemployment and underemployment as well as the overrepresentation of people of color in jobs that offer no health coverage limits the access of Blacks and Latinos to adequate health care

(Blendon et al. 1989; Council on Ethical and Judicial Affairs, 1990). National data show that Blacks and Latinos are less likely than Whites to be insured. For example, of non-Hispanic Whites, 18.6% were uninsured for all or part of 1987, as were 29.8% of Blacks and 41.4% of Latinos (Short, Monheit, and Beauregard 1989; Short 1990). Often because of people of color's employment situation, many cannot afford to miss time from work to obtain medical care, so many enter the health care system at a point when their condition is advanced. This often requires a longer and more expensive hospital stay; in some cases, later detection often means poorer survival rates (Munoz 1988; Morris et al. 1989). Yet, there is a cyclical effect between being poor and health; that is, being poor often leads to poor health status, which tends to diminish earning capabilities, which contributes to poorer health (Dutton 1994). Other barriers to health care are cultural and language factors, especially for Latinos and other immigrant groups. Latinos often cite differences in culture and language as reasons for not practicing preventive care (Vega and Amaro 1994). According to Chang and Fortier (1998), in 1990 almost 32 million U.S. residents older than age 5 (about 14% of the population) spoke a language other than English at home. More than half of these non-English speakers (17 million) spoke Spanish, and other common languages were French, German, Italian, and Chinese (Chang and Fortier 1998). In addition, although Latinos constitute approximately 9% of the U.S. population according to the 1990 Census, less than 5% of all U.S. physicians and medical school students are Latinos (Vega and Amaro 1994; Council on Scientific Affairs 1991). The provider's familiarity with the patient's culture and language can foster a better doctor–patient relationship and affect the quality of health service received (Chang and Fortier 1998). Language is important because Latinos who speak English are more likely to have a regular source of medical care compared to those who speak only Spanish (Council on Scientific Affairs 1991). In addition, Latinos who are less assimilated (or acculturated) into U.S. society are less likely to seek medical attention and more likely to treat their illnesses using folk medicine or seeking folk healers (Anderson et al. 1981).

Overall, non-Whites tend to report higher levels of dissatisfaction with the quality of care they receive (Council on Ethical and Judicial Affairs 1990). Racial and ethnic minority populations often access medical care in non-optimal settings, and due to their health coverage, or lack thereof, people of color are more likely to seek medical attention at hospital emergency rooms or other organized care settings where they are likely to see a different provider at each visit (Blendon et al. 1989). Thus, Latinos and Blacks are more likely than Whites not to have a regular physician who provides primary and regular care. Because Latinos and Blacks tend to seek medical care at the emergency room they are also more likely to wait longer to receive care (Blendon et al. 1989; Council on Ethical and Judicial Affairs 1990). It is easy to understand why the lack of continuity in health care and time spent waiting to receive health care are sources for dissatisfaction.

Perceived racial differences and discrimination also affect the quality of medical care, treatment, and medical procedures available to Whites versus non-Whites. The Council of Ethical and Judicial Affairs (1990) of the American Medical Association examined Black and White health disparities. They found that after controlling for health insurance, income, and clinical status, Whites are more likely to receive coronary angiography, bypass surgery, angioplasty, chemodialysis, intensive care for pneumonia, and kidney transplants than Blacks. This suggests that Blacks are less likely to have access to these kinds of medical treatments than Whites, economic reasons aside. Further, when Blacks are recommended to receive transplants they are more likely to wait longer than Whites (Sullivan 1991).

Satisfaction and quality of care are also influenced by the treatment patients receive at the doctor's office. For example, in the case of a non-English-speaking patient an interpreter often mediates the relationship with the doctor. It is not uncommon that when a non-English-speaking patient goes to see a doctor that anyone who is bilingual, such as an employee, family member (e.g., a child), or a friend, serves as an interpreter (Torres 1998). Typically, these individuals have no formal interpretation training. This can contribute to inaccuracies and to the inability of a patient to feel free to disclose important, personal, and relevant information. It is difficult to receive good quality health care when fundamental patient rights are violated when language barriers exist. Language barriers have also been found to play a role in compliance with medical recommendations and with continuation of treatment (Estrada, Trevino, and Ray 1990).

Evidence of systematic bias in medical care continues to accumulate. For example, Schulman et al. (1999) found that race and sex of patient independently influence how physicians manage chest pain. These researchers found that women and Blacks were less likely to be referred for cardiac cauterization than men and Whites, after adjusting for symptoms, the physicians' estimates of probability of coronary disease, and clinical characteristics. And Black women, overall, were least likely to be referred to cauterization. These findings are consistent with other epidemiological studies that report that differences in treatment exist according to race and sex (Carlisle, Leake, and Shapiro 1997; Ayanian and Epstein 1991; Wenneker and Epstein 1989). Williams and Rucker (in press) have recently argued that unconscious discrimination lies at the foundation of these differences in medical treatment and have outlined multiple strategies to address it.

Participation in Medical Research

The participation of people of color (irrespective of gender) in medical research studies is important for several reasons. First, as noted earlier, there is a disparity in health outcomes between Whites and non-Whites. Second, recruitment of people of color can directly contribute to the accuracy of estimating disease prevalence within and between groups, including gender (Welsh et al. 1994; Krieger et al. 1993). Medical research should also consider recruiting equal numbers of men and women of color; it is important to investigate how risk factors and diseases influence the health of men and women of color (Krieger et al. 1993). Finally, possible ethnic differences in metabolism of pharmacological agents need to be observed to ensure the safety and efficacy of new drugs for all individuals (Brawley and Tejeda 1995). Given that the biological characteristics of a social group are influenced by the habitual behaviors of that group in response to the constraints of its environment (Jackson 1992), observed biological differences can reflect the adaptation of racial groups to their environmental conditions.

Although there is a need for people of color to participate as subjects in medical and clinical studies, two major reasons are often cited for the low representation of people of color. First, because it is often assumed that research findings on White males are generalizable and applicable to other populations, ethnic minorities have been actively excluded from recruitment for participation. Second, when people of color are recruited to participate they are less likely to consent, largely due to distrust (Brawley and Tejeda 1995). Communities of color tend to distrust government medical institutions because there is a history of using them for medical experimentation.

Fears of exploitation by the medical profession by Blacks date back to the antebellum period when slaves and free Blacks were used as subjects for dissection and medical experiments (Gamble 1997). We note two examples from the antebellum period. Dr. Thomas Hamilton used a slave to test remedies for heatstroke by subjecting his subject to sit nude in a pit that had been heated to a high temperature, where only the subject's head was above ground. The goal of the experiment was to find a remedy that would make it possible for masters to force their slaves to work longer hours during the hottest days of the year (Boney 1967). Similarly, Dr. J. Marion Sims, the father of modern gynecology, used three slave women to develop an operation to repair vesicovaginal fistulas. He performed surgery on one of these women 30 times during a four-year period. After he had perfected the procedure using slave women, he attempted it with anesthesia on White women (Sims 1889; Gamble 1997). However, the best documented and widely known racially biased government-sponsored health experiment against Blacks is the Tuskegee Syphilis Study (1932 to 1972). Its primary objective was to follow the natural progression of syphilis in approximately 400 Black men who were diagnosed with the disease compared to a control group of 200 uninfected men (Jones 1981). These men were never treated for syphilis, although penicillin was already an accepted treatment for the disease.

An expanded role for the participation of people of color in health research must extend beyond the role of subject. Participation should be viewed more broadly to include people of color as investigators, analysts, and policy makers (Spigner 1994).

Practical Guidelines for Assessing Race

Although we have argued that race is not primarily biological, it is nonetheless an important construct in health-related research. There are several fundamental reasons why studying race is important. First, if race is perceived to be "real," then it is real in its consequences (Thomas 1928). That is, the established racial and ethnic categories capture an important aspect of the inequalities and injustices embedded in the U.S. social structure (See and Wilson 1988). Health outcomes reflect, at least in part, the differentials in power and status between groups.

Second, racial categories have historically reflected racism. As discussed previously, racism is an ideology of superiority that justifies the subjugation, exploitation, and domination of groups that are defined as genetically or culturally inferior (Krieger et al. 1993; See and Wilson 1988). As such, in the U.S., racial categories capture the racial subordination and the system of power affording Whites domination over non-White groups and the unequal access of people of color to limited resources. Racism as an ideology has had a great influence on residential segregation, quality of education, labor participation, access to political office, inter-racial marriages, and health (Bobo, Kluegel, and Smith 1997).

Third, how racial categories are constructed has an effect on all aspects of daily lives of the groups. For example, it is not uncommon for non-Whites to endure racism in the form of daily hassles that include insults and demeaning treatment by Whites (Forman, Williams, and Jackson 1997). These experiences of discrimination adversely affect health and play a role in accounting for racial differentials in disease (Williams et al. 1997; Krieger 1999).

Fourth, race is a fundamental organizing principle in our society and it is central to identity formation (Omi and Winant 1994). An understanding of a shared history and common experiences stemming from immigration, discrimination, residential segregation, and occupational status and context often provides the basis for group solidarity and is manifested in lifestyle and struggles for limited resources (Williams 1997).

Current efforts to monitor the health status and well-being of groups of people within the United States include collecting and reporting data on racial and ethnic groups, but these methods of data collection are inadequate, stemming from the increasing diversity of the U.S. We make the following recommendations adopted from Williams (1999a):

1. There is a continuing need for uniform assessment of race and ethnicity by government-administered health surveys, as well as by the wider research community. Researchers need to move beyond a simple Black/White dichotomy and include other groups in their studies. Given the heterogeneity of the U.S., there is a critical need for the inclusion of identifiers for such groups as Asians and Latinos, as well as for the major subgroups of these categories. Researchers should use terms that are broadly recognized by a variety of people and that reflect the preferences of respondents. In addition, we recommend that identifiers be included to explore the heterogeneity within the White and Black population. In this fashion some of the uniqueness of these various groups can be explored.

2. Racial/ethnic data should be routinely utilized in the design, implementation, and evaluation of health studies and health programs. There tends to be inadequate data, especially morbidity data, for American Indians, Latinos, and Asian subgroups. Standard sampling strategies and designs fail to capture a representative number of these groups because of geographical distribution and potentially small numbers in the general population. Reliable estimates for the distribution of disease are often unavailable; hence, analysis of heterogeneity within a given racial group is unavailable.

3. Questionnaires should be translated and measurement instruments should be culturally appropriate. Often health researchers do not translate study instru-

ments into other languages, thus limiting their sample to those who have a proficiency in the English language. Researchers should also ensure that their new study instruments meet the test of conceptual, scale, and norm equivalence. Conceptual equivalence refers to similarities in the meaning of the concepts used in the assessment. Scale equivalence is the use of questionnaire items that are familiar to all groups, while norm equivalence ensures that the norms developed for the targeted group are appropriate and not arbitrarily assigned from another population.

4. Communication mechanisms should be built in conjunction with racial/ethnic communities to ensure that they receive findings from current studies and have input in future research and interventions.

5. Whenever racial/ethnic data are reported, more attention should be given to interpretation. Researchers need to indicate why race/ethnicity is being used, the limitations of racial/ethnic data, and how findings should be interpreted. The presentation of data on racial differences should routinely stratify them by socioeconomic status within racial groups. Failure to do this may misspecify complex health risks and may have unintended social consequences.

6. Studies of race and health should be abandoned in favor of studies that identify racial factors that influence health outcomes. For example, information that provides a broader context should be collected. This includes a better assessment of socioeconomic status and wealth, and economic and non-economic dimensions of discrimination. In addition to the aforementioned, data such as nativity, acculturation, and years since migration are key factors to understanding the health status of immigrants.

7. In studying race and health, gender should not be ignored. Often being a woman and being of color means that relevant intersections and complexities are ignored, especially as they relate to women's health. In this country, gender often translates into research on White women, and race means research on men of color; researchers need to be sensitive to this cleavage. A better understanding of the questions regarding the current health and mental health status of women of color in the United States is much needed. It is important to understand how economic circumstances, employment, stress, poor nutrition, poor sanitation, inadequate housing, family strains, motherhood, and the role of physical, emotional, and sexual abuse influence women of color's health. Gender should not be merely a variable in the data researchers collect. Rather, the consideration of women of color and their health status should flow from a strong research agenda that cuts across all of the recommendations listed above.

The challenge for the scientific community is to move away from traditional ways of researching race and health and to develop new tools and methods of analysis. Yet researchers should keep in mind that the legacy of the past—of conquest, slavery, exclusion, and removal—continues to shape the present. Historical and prevailing attitudes, conceptions, and beliefs about race govern social policy and social arrangements that limit the access to health care and the well-being of people of color. This legacy also reveals that the health outcomes of different racial and eth-nic groups are part of the socio-historical and political process in which race cate-gories are created, transformed, changed, and ultimately destroyed.

References

Adler NE, Boyce T, Chesney MA, Folkman S, Syme SL. Socioeconomic Inequalities in Health: No Easy Solution. JAMA. 1993;269:3140–3145.

Anderson M, Feinberg SE. Black, white, and shades of gray (and brown and yellow). Chance. 1995;8(1):15–18.

Anderson MJ. The American Census: A Social History. New Haven: Yale University Press; 1988.

Anderson RM, Lewis SZ, Giachello AL, Chiu G. Access to Medical Care Among Hispanic Population of the Southwestern United States. J Health Soc Behav. 1981;22:78-89.

Antonovsky A. Social Class, Life Expectancy, and Overall Mortality. Milbank Memorial Fund Quarterly. 1967;45:31-73.

Ayanian JZ, Epstein AM. Differences in the Use of Procedures Between Women and Men Hospitalized for Coronary Heart Disease. N Engl J Med. 1991;325:221-5.

Ballard R. The Construction of a Conceptual Vision: 'Ethnic Groups' and the 1991 UK Census. Ethnic and Racial Studies. 1997;20:82-194.

Barrera M. Race and Class in the Southwest: A Theory of Racial Inequality. Notre Dame: University of Notre Dame Press; 1979.

Bauman K. Direct measures of poverty as indicators of economic need: evidence from the survey of income and program participation. U.S. Census Bureau Population Division Technical Working Paper No. 30; 1998.

Blendon RJ, Aiken LH, Freeman HE, Corey CR. Access to Medical Care for Blacks and White Americans: A Matter of Continuing Concern. JAMA. 1989;261:278-281.

Bobo L, Kluegel JR, Smith RA. Laissez-Faire Racism: The Crystallization of Kinder, Gentle, and Antiblack Ideology. In: Tuch SA, Martin J, eds. Racial Attitudes in the 1990s: Continuity and Change. Westport, Conn: Praeger; 1997.

Bobo L, Zubrinsky CL. Attitudes on residential integration: Perceived status differences, mere in-group preference, or racial prejudice? Soc Forces.1996;74(3):883-909.

Boney FN. Doctor Thomas Hamilton: Two Views on a Gentleman of the Old South. Phylon 1967;28:288-292.

Bonilla-Silva E. Rethinking racism: toward a structural interpretation. Am Soc Rev. 1996;62:465-480.

Brandt AM. Racism and research: the case of the Tuskegee Syphilis Study. Hastings Cent Rep. 1978;8(6):21-29.

Brawley OW, Tejeda, H. Minority Inclusion in Clinical Trials: Issues and Potential Strategies. In: Journal of the National Cancer Institute Monographs. 1995;17:55-57.

Bunker, JP, Gomby DS, Kehrer B, eds. Pathways to Health: The Role of Social Factors. Menlo Park, Calif.: Henry J. Kaiser Family Foundation; 1989.

Carlisle DM, Leake BD, Shapiro MF. Racial and Ethnic Disparities in the use of Cardiovascular Pro-cedures: Associations with Type of Health Insurance. Am J Public Health. 1997;87:263-7.

Chang PH, Fortier JP. Language Barriers to Health Care: An Overview. J Health Care Poor Underserved. 1998;9:S5-S20.

Cole RE, Deskins Jr. DR. Racial factors in site location and employment patterns of Japanese auto firms in America. Calif Mgmt Rev. 1988;31(1):9-22.

Cooper RS. A note on the biologic concept of race and its application in epidemiologic research. Am Heart J. 1984;108(3):715-723.

Council on Ethical and Judicial Affairs. Black-White Disparities in Health Care. JAMA. 1990; 263:2344-46.

Council on Scientific Affairs. Hispanic Health in the United States. JAMA. 1991;265:248-252.

Cox OC. Caste, Class, and Race. New York: Doubleday; 1948.

Davis JA, Smith TW. General Social Survey, 1972-1990 NORC. Chicago: National Opinion Research Center; 1990.

Devine PG. Prejudice and out-group perception. In: Tesser A. Adv Soc Psychol. 1995:467-524.

Duster T. A Social Frame for Biological Knowledge. In Duster, T and Garrett K eds. *Cultural Perspectives on Biological Knowledge*. Norwood, NJ: Ablex Publishing: 1984.

Dutton DB. Social Class, Health, and Illness. In: Schwartz HD. *Dominant Issues in Medical Sociology*. New York: McGraw-Hill; 1994.

Economic Report of the President. Washington, D.C.: U.S. Government Printing Office; 1998.

Eller TJ. *Household Wealth and Asset Ownership: 1991. U.S. Bureau of the Census, Current Population Reports, P70-34*. Washington, D.C.: U.S. Government Printing Office; 1994.

Engels F. *The Condition of the Working Class in English*. New York: Oxford University Press; 1993.

Estrada AL, Trevino F, Ray LA. Health Care Utilization Barriers Among Mexican Americans: Evidence from HHANES 1982-1984. *Am J Public Health*. 1990;80:27S-31S.

Evinger S. How shall we measure our nation's diversity? *Chance*. 1995;8(1):7-14.

Fix M, Struyk RJ. *Clear and Convincing Evidence: Measurement of Discrimination in America*. Washington, D.C.: Urban Institute Press; 1993.

Forman TA, Williams DR, Jackson JS. Race, Place, and Discrimination. *Soc Problems*. 1997;9:231-261.

Gamble VN. Under the Shadow of Tuskegee: African Americans and Health Care. *Am J Public Health*. 1997;87:1773-1778.

Giles E, Elliot O. Race Identification from Cranial Measurements. *J Forensic Sci*. 1962;7: 147-157.

Goodman AH. Bred in the Bones? *Sciences*. 1997;37:20-5.

Gould SJ. *Ever Since Darwin*. New York: W.W. Norton; 1977

Hahn RA. The state of federal health statistics on racial and ethnic groups. *JAMA*. 1992;267(2):268-271.

Hilton JL, von Hippel W. Stereotypes. *Annu Rev Psychol*. 1996;47:237-271.

Hummer RA, Rogers RG, Nam CB, LeClere FB. Race/Ethnicity, Nativity, and U.S. Adult Mortality. *Soc Sci Q*. 1999;80:136-153.

Jackson FL. Race and ethnicity as biological constructs. *Ethn Dis*. 1992;2:120-125.

Jary D, Jary J. *Collins Dictionary of Sociology*. Glaslow, Scotland: Harper Collins; 1991.

Jaynes GD, Williams RM. *A common destiny: Blacks and American Society*. Washington D.C.: National Accademy Press; 1989.

Jensen AR. How Much Can We Boost IQ and Scholastic Achievement? *Harvard Educ Rev*. 1969;Winter: 1-123.

Jones JH. *Bad Blood: The Tuskegee Syphilis Experiment*. New York: The Free Press; 1981.

Jordan WD. *White Over Black: American Attitudes Toward the Negro, 1550-1812*. Baltimore: Penguin Books; 1968.

Kirschenman J, Neckerman KM. We'd love to hire them, but...: the meaning of race for employers. In: Jencks C, Peterson PE, eds. *The Urban Underclass*. Washington, D.C.: The Brookings Institution; 1991:203-232.

Kralt, JM. Ethnic Origin In the Canadian Census, 1871-1981. In: Petryshyn WR, ed. *Changing Realities: Social Trends Among Ukrainian Canadians*. Edmonton: The Canadian Institute for Ukrainian Studies; 1980.

Krieger N, Bassett M. The health of black folk: Disease, class, and ideology in science. *Monthly Rev*. 1986;38(3):74-85.

Krieger N. Embodying Inequality: A Review of Concepts, Measures, and Methods for Studying Health Consequences of Discrimination. *Int J Health Serv*. 1999;29(2):295-352.

Krieger N. Shades of difference: Theoretical underpinnings of the medical controversy on black/white differences in the United States, 1830-1870. *Int J Health Serv*. 1987;17:259-278.

Krieger N, Rowley DL, Herman AA, Avery B, Phillips MT. Racism, Sexism, and Social Class: Implications for Studies of Health, Disease, and Well-being. *Am J Prev Med*. 1993;9:82-122.

Last JM, ed. *A Dictionary of Epidemiology, 3rd Ed*. New York: Oxford University Press; 1995.

LaVeist TA. Beyond dummy variables and sample selection: What health services researchers ought to know about race as a variable. *Health Serv Res*. 1994;29:1-16.

Lee SE. Racial Classifications in the U.S. Census: 1890-1990. *Ethnic Racial Stud*. 1993;16:75-94.

Lewontin RC. *Biology as Ideology: The Doctrine of DNA*. New York: Harper Perennial; 1991.

Lieberson S. *A Piece of the Pie: Black and White Immigrants since 1880*. Berkeley: University of California Press; 1980.

Lillie-Blanton M, Parsons PE, Gayle H, Dievler A. Racial Differentials in Health: Not Just Black and White, but Shades of Gray. *Annu Rev Public Health*. 1996;17:411-48.

Littlefield A, Lieberman L, Reynolds LT. Redefining Race: The Potential Demise of a Concept in Physical Anthropology. *Curr Anthropol.* 1982;23:641-647.

Marmot MG, Smith GD, Stansfeld S, Patel C, North F, Head J, White I, Brunner E, Feeney A. Health Inequalities Among British Civil Servants: The Whitehall II Study. *Lancet.* 1991;337: 1387-93.

Massey DA, Gross AB, Shibuya K. Migration, segregation, and the geographic concentration of poverty. *Am Soc Rev.* 1994;59:425-445.

Massey DS. The age of extremes: concentrated affluence and poverty in the twenty-first century. *Demography.* 1996;33:395-428.

Montagu A. *Man's Most Dangerous Myth: The Fallacy of Race.* New York: The World Publishing Co.; 1964.

Morris DL, Lucero GT, Joyce EV, Hannigan EV, Tucker ER. Cervical Cancer, A Major Killer of Hispanic Women: Implications for Health Education. *Health Educ.* 1989;20:23-28.

Muir DE. Race: The Myth of Racism. *Sociol Inquiry.* 1993;63:339-350.

Munoz E. Care for the Hispanic Poor: A Growing Segment of American Society. *JAMA.* 1988; 260:2711-2712.

National Center for Health Statistics. *Health, United States, 1998 Health and Aging Chartbook.* Hyattsville, Md.: USDHHS. 1999.

Navarro V. Race or Classes Versus Race and Class: Growing Mortality Differentials in the United States. *Int J Health Serv.* 1991;21:229-235.

Neckerman KM, Kirschenman J. Hiring strategies, racial bias, and inner-city workers. *Soc Problems.* 1991;38:433-447.

Oliver ML, Shapiro TM. *Black Wealth/White Wealth.* New York: Routledge; 1995.

Omi M, Winant H. *Racial Formation in the United States: From the 1960s to the 1990s.* New York: Routledge; 1994.

Pryor E, Goldmann GJ, Royce DA. Future Issues for the Census of Canada. *Int Migration Rev.* 1991;25:167-75.

Sampson RJ, Wilson WJ. Toward a theory of race, crime, and urban inequality. In: Hagan J, Peterson RD, eds. *Crime and Inequality.* Stanford, Calif.: Stanford University Press; 1995:37-54.

Schulman KA, et al. The Effect of Race and Sex on Physicians' Recommendations for Cardiac Catheterization. *N Engl J Med.* 1999;340:618-26.

See KO, Wilson WJ. Race and Ethnicity. In: Smelser NJ, ed. *Handbook of Sociology.* Beverly Hills, Calif.: Sage Publications; 1988.

Seymour-Smith C, ed. *Macmillan Dictionary of Anthropology.* London: Macmillan; 1986.

Sharpe R. In latest recession, only blacks suffered net employment loss. *Wall Street Journal.* 1993;LXXIV(233).

Short PF, Monheit AC, Beauregard K. *National Medical Expenditure Survey: Estimates of the Uninsured Americans: Research Findings I.* Rockville, Md.: National Center for Health Services Research and Health Care Technology Assessment; 1989.

Short PF. *National Medical Expenditure Survey: Estimates of the Uninsured Population, Calendar Year 1987; Data Summary 2.* Rockville, Md.: National Center for Health Services Research and Health Care Technology Assessment; 1990.

Shuman H, Steeh C, Bobo L, Krysan M. *Racial Attitudes in America: Trends and Interpretations. Revised Edition.* Cambridge, Mass.: Harvard University Press; 1997.

Sims JM. *The Story of My Life.* New York: Appleton; 1889.

Singh GK, Yu SM. Adverse Pregnancy Outcomes: Differences between U.S. and Foreign-Born Women in Major U.S. Racial and Ethnic Groups. *Am J Public Health.* 1996;86:837-843.

Smelser N, Wilson, WJ, Mitchell F, eds. *America Becoming: Racial Trends and Their Consequences.* Vols. I and II. National Academies Press; 2001.

Spigner C. Black Participation in Health Research: A Functionalist Overview. *J Health Educ.* 1994;25:210-214.

Sullivan LW. Effects of Discrimination and Racism on Access to Health Care. *JAMA.* 1991;266:2674.

Thomas WI, Thomas DS. *The Child in America: Behavior Problems and Programs.* New York: A.A. Knopf; 1928.

Torres RE. The Pervading Role of Language on Health. *J Health Care for the Poor and Underserved.* 1998;9:S21-S25.

Tucker C, Kojetin B. Testing Racial and Ethnic Origin Questions in the CPS Supplement. *Monthly Labor Rev.* 1996;119:3-7.

Turner RJ, Wheaton B, Lloyd DA. The Epidemiology of Social Stress. *Am Soc Rev.* 1995;60:104-125.

U.S. Bureau of the Census. *Income by Educational Attainment for Persons 18 Years Old and Over, by Age, Sex, Race, and Hispanic Origin: March 1996, Current Population Report.* Washington, D.C.: U.S. Government Printing Office; 1997.

Vega W, Amaro H. Latino Outlook: Good Health, Uncertain Prognosis. *Ann Rev Public Health.* 1994;15:39-67.

Welsh KA, Ballard E, Nash F, Raiford K, Harrell L. Issues Affecting Minority Participation in Research Studies of Alzheimer Disease. *Alzheimer Dis Assoc Disord.* 1994;8: 38-48.

Wenneker MB, Epstein AM. Racial Inequalities in the Use of Procedures for Patients with Ischemic Heart Disease in Massachusetts. *JAMA.* 1989;261:253-7.

Williams DR. The Monitoring of Racial/Ethnic Status in the USA: Data Quality Issues. *Ethnicity and Health.* 1999a;4:121-137.

Williams DR. Race, Socioeconomic Status, and Health: The Added Effect of Racism and Discrimination. *Ann N Y Acad Sci.* 1999b;896:173-188.

Williams DR. Race and Health: Basic Questions, Emerging Directions. *Ann Epidemiol.* 1997;7: 322-333.

Willaims DR. Race/Ethnicity and Socioeconomic Status: Measurement and Methodological Issues. *Int J Health Services.* 1996;26:483-505.

Williams DR. Racism and Health: A Research Agenda. *Ethnicity and Disease.* 1990;6:1-6.

Williams DR, Collins C. U.S. Socioeconomic and Racial Differences in Health. *Annu Rev Sociol.* 1995;21:349-86.

Williams DR, Rucker TD. Racial and Ethnic disparities in Healthcare: A Conceptual Framework and Research Directions. *Healthcare Financing Review* (under review).

Williams DR, Jackson JS, Brown TN, Torres M, Forman TA, Brown K. Traditional and Contemporary Prejudice and Urban Whites' Support for Affirmative Action and Government Help. *Soc Problems.* 1999;46(4):1–25.

Williams DR, Yu Y, Jackson J, Anderson N. Racial differences in physical and mental health: socioeconomic status, stress, and discrimination. *J Health Psychol.* 1997;2(3):335–351.

Wright CD. *The History and Growth of the United States Census.* Washington, D.C.: Government Printing Office; 1966.

Chapter 2

PHYSICAL ANTHROPOLOGY: THE QUESTION *of* RACE *and* PHYSICAL VARIATION

Douglas H. Ubelaker, PhD

R ace concepts pervade American thought and affect many aspects of daily life. Each day, the media bombards us with "racial" perspectives on significant events and most Americans think of themselves and others as being members of various racial groups. These social classifications can extend into science and affect the manner in which data are collected and interpreted. This chapter explores the history of race concepts, especially as they relate to human physical variation and physical anthropology. The goal of this discussion is to provide a framework for assessing how these concepts affect health studies.

Early Classification

Much of scientific nomenclature can be traced back to the 18th century work of the Swedish botanist Carl [von] Linné (Carolus Linnaeus, 1707–1778). His binomial system applied to comparative studies designates humans as a single species, *Homo sapiens*. Within the species, he suggested that four geographical subdivisions could be recognized: American (*H. americanus*), European (*H. europaeus*), African (*H. afer*), and Asiatic (*H. asiaticus*) (Barnouw 1989; Brøberg 1997). His groupings were geographical and group descriptions concentrated on skin color and behavior attributes. A subsequent classification by Johann Friedrich Blumenbach (1752–1840) added a Malayan category (Barnouw 1989; Kelso 1974) to those proposed by Linnaeus. In an attempt to inject more science into the racial typology, Blumenbach added anatomical features, primarily of the head.

These early efforts at human nomenclature were framed from a largely religious perspective on the assumption that a natural order of human grouping existed, waiting to be discovered and described, and that these categories were relatively unchanging (Kelso 1974). Subsequent attempts at classification varied enormously in the number of groups differentiated and reflected the tendency of the classifiers to be either "lumpers" or "splitters." For example, Morton and Hrdlicka tended to regard American Indians as belonging to a single group whereas Retzius, Meigs, Virchow, Ten Kate, Dixon, and Hooton all inclined to classify them into various subgroups (Stewart and Newman 1951).

With evolutionary theory came the understanding of the role that natural selection may have played in producing human diversity. Laden with the typology and nomenclature of their predecessors, scholars with an evolutionary perspective struggled to document human diversity and explain it through regional adaptation. Examples include Carleton Coon's exhaustive work (e.g., 1962, 1965) describing physical characteristics of peoples around the world and his attempt to trace modern diversity back into the fossil record.

Increasingly, scholars developed difficulty in adequately fitting human diversity into any of the various racial categories and explaining it in terms of evolutionary principles. As physical anthropologists set about documenting phenotypic and, more recently, genetic variation throughout the world, the boundaries of the "types" began to become very blurred. The concepts of races being "static" or "pure" evolved into more dynamic definitions. For example, in 1941, *Webster's New International Dictionary of the English Language* defined "race" as "the descendants of a common ancestor, a family, tribe, people, or nation believed or presumed to belong to the same stock." A footnote adds "A 'race' is not a permanent entity, something static, it is dynamic and is slowly developing and changing," quoting Roland B. Dixon. Other definitions include "state of being one of a special people or ethnical stock" and "a group or assemblage of organisms exhibiting general similarities but not sufficiently distinct from other forms to constitute a species."

Controversy over Terminology

The old type concepts were also laden with value judgements and racism that were products of their times. Concepts of "racial purity" were ripe for political exploitation and misuse, as was witnessed through the monstrous actions of Hitler and the Third Reich from 1933 to 1945 (Spencer 1997). The tarnished history of the race concept and the diverse associations that had become linked with it led some anthropologists to suggest that it should be abandoned. For example, in 1942, Ashley Montagu suggested that the existence of races was a myth, and a dangerous one at that because of its potential for misuse. Stewart (1944) countered that the study of race should be separated from racism, and that there was still a need to document human diversity, but he admitted that the word "race" was becoming difficult to define consistently.

Through all of this, the old concepts of races as fixed, pure types that could be ranked in various ways were largely discarded. The need to document and understand human diversity persisted, however. In 1956, Boyd pointed out how race concepts (or the lack of them) varied in different cultures. By that time, scientific studies were documenting how no specific attribute could define a grouping because of the inherent variation within human populations.

In 1962, Garn discussed human diversity in terms of geographical, local, and micro races but noted the variance of opinion on terminology. Others, following Montagu (1964), dropped the term "race" in favor of more neutral terms such as "ethnic group" to discuss human variation. The terms "breeding population" and "cline" (Brace 1995a, Brace et al. 1993) also have been substituted in discussions of regional population variation.

In spite of growing uneasiness with racial terminology, it continued to be used among many anthropologists and other students of human diversity, perhaps out of a combination of tradition and lack of universally accepted alternative terminology. For example, in Osborne's 1971 edited volume *The Biological and Social Meaning of Race*, W. W. Howells defines race as "the variation of populations within a typical animal species (Howells 1971, p. 3). In another chapter, Dobzhansky defines races as "populations which differ in frequency, or in prevalence, of some genes" (1971, p. 18). Elsewhere, Damon cautions that despite the terminological difficulties and past and potential future misuse of the race concept, it remains important to study "group differences in disease and serves to benefit the health care of all people" (Damon 1971, p. 57).

For King in 1971, race concept became "an attempt to describe the manner in which individual variation within and between populations is related to heredity, development, and environment." King's writing shows respect for the important role culture plays in shaping population definitions and history.

Writing in 1974, Kelso asked the rhetorical question, "if racial terminology is so controversial, why use it?" His answer was "they continue to be useful in providing a broad range of background information on the distribution of human variation, and also as a basis for determining the effects that might be due to long-term geographical isolation" (Kelso 1974, p. 310). Kelso added that races are not "self-evident, natural units," but simply ways of "dividing up human variation."

Two years later, Lasker (1976) distinguished "biological race" from "social race," noting that membership in the former is "membership by descent." The "descent" component in race also was emphasized in Krantz' 1980 discussion that most anthropologists define human races as those who form a breeding population or gene pool; have similar inherited biological characteristics; and share these traits from a common ancestral type (Krantz 1980, p. 17). However, Krantz noted that these three components "do not coincide at all on a theoretical level, and on a practical level they agree only sometimes." Krantz suggests it is more useful to distinguish between "climatic races" and "descent groups."

Within forensic anthropology, scholars attempt to identify the "race" of an individual from skeletonized remains in an effort to assist law enforcement to identify unknown individuals. Commenting on this intellectual effort, Stewart cautioned that whereas in the original zoological sense, the term referred to a subdivision of a species based on appearance (phenotype), the term now "means different things to different people" (Stewart 1979, p. 227). Stewart also recognized the social dimensions of public race concepts in adding "from the stand point of forensic anthropology, it is necessary to categorize the skeletal remains of unknowns in terms that reflect racial reality as locally understood" (Stewart 1979, p. 227).

An overview of race discussion by Barnouw in 1989 concluded "many physical anthropologists therefore believe that the concept of cline is more useful for research purposes than the race concept" (Barnouw 1989, p. 40).

Another overview at about the same time by Relethford (1990, p. 148) assembled data of variation in skin color as measured by mean skin reflectance. These data revealed lighter skin color in South African Blacks than among the Guarani Indians of Brazil, the Aguarana Indians of Peru, the Mahar group of India, the Bareng Paroja group of Indian, a population from New Guinea, and the Garifuna of Belize. The point here is that a single attribute, even one as important to "race" classification as skin color, cannot separate populations from a particular geographic area.

Unfortunately, these old arguments have not been resolved. The emotional debates about race terminology following World War II led to reduced discussion until relatively recently, but within the last few years, anthropologists have begun renewed discussion of the issues involved. For the most part, this discussion has been welcomed to clarify thinking on this important topic (Gill 1998). Appropriately, much of this discussion has involved social anthropologists as the social dimensions of terminology and the social factors shaping human diversity increasingly are recognized. This discussion has revealed the complexity of the issues involved and the need for sharpened terminology.

Surveys of Scholarly Opinion

Current literature fails to document that groups of humans can be found anywhere on the globe displaying physical characteristics that distinguish them completely from others; we are all one species with some internal variation. Nevertheless, some scholars continue to feel that a typological approach is useful to view this variation in a comparative context. Others are focused in problem-oriented research that does not require such an approach. Lieberman (1997), for example, reports on a survey of PhD-granting departments in 1984–1985 regarding agreement with the statement: "There are biological races in the species *Homo sapiens*." Majority agreement was found in biology departments and among males in biological anthropology. Less support for the statement was found among female biological anthropologists and within groups of cultural anthropology, psychological anthropology, and developmental psychology.

Cartmill (1999) reports a survey of language relating to racial typology in papers published in *American Anthropologist*. He not only reports continued use of the terminology but was unable to detect a significant temporal trend in use within the last 30 years.

Human Origins

Discussion of issues relevant to this topic have been stimulated by recent debate within paleoanthropology on human origins. Discussion has focused on whether the extent of current human variation is a relatively new development or if similar variation has characterized the human species since its formation (Mellars and Stringer 1989; Wolpoff and Caspari 1997). Workers on all sides of this issue refer to human variation in the general sense and not to specific "racial" groups.

Forensic Applications

Research in forensic anthropology has continued to improve techniques of esti-mating "race" from human remains (Burris and Harris 1998; Byers, Churchill, and Curran 1997; Craig 1995; Gill 1995; Gill and Rhine 1990). Progress in this area includes a sophisticated multivariate computer technique derived from measure-ments taken on identified forensic cases and related museum collections (Ousley and Jantz 1996).

Some forensic anthropologists substitute the terms "ancestry" or "ethnic group" to avoid possible reference to a typological race concept. Kennedy (1995) has dis-cussed the line walked by forensic anthropologists in this area of study and the com-plexity he has experienced teaching both forensic anthropology and the dynamics of human variation at the university level. Sauer (1992, 1993) and Ubelaker (1996), have argued that in estimating "racial" affiliation for law enforcement, most foren-sic anthropologists are not revealing a Blumenbach-like classification of world pop-ulations but rather attempting to determine how the person would have been regard-ed by the communities in which they lived. This position recognizes the social dimensions of current public race classifications. While heavily influenced by his-torical and social forces, the groups do display some physical differences that allow forensic determinations to be made with varying degrees of confidence. The impor-tant point here is that forensic anthropologists are not looking at human variation and assigning typological categories. Instead, they recognize that, especially in American society, many individuals consider themselves and/or are considered by their communities to belong to particular "racial groups." This view recognizes that public race concepts are not dependent upon scientific analysis but are based in folk culture shaped by social and historical factors. Analysis can suggest ancestral origins (Brace 1995b) and from that process social classification of "race."

Cultural Factors

The social component in race categories within America has recently become an active topic among social anthropologists and related scholars (American Anthropological Association 1998; Gregory and Sanjek 1994; Harrison 1998; Keita and Kittles 1997; Mukhopadhyay and Moses 1997; Paredes 1997; Smedley 1999; Templeton 1999; Visweswaran 1998). While some have argued that the term "race" should be abandoned because of its history of use and misuse, others note that study of the terms and people grouped under the terms offers an opportunity to critical-ly examine important aspects of society (Baker 1998; Harrison 1998; Studstill 1998).

Race in Health Science

As noted by Overfield (1995), many health-related conditions vary by sex and pop-ulation. Recognition of sex and ancestry of the patient may alert the physician to consider conditions that are of increased probability. Like forensic anthropologists, medical workers are to some extent bound to the existing racial terminology since much of the available literature is presented using this language and many patients label themselves with "racial" affiliation.

Health workers should realize, however, the great variation in the use of racial terminology. As noted throughout this essay, racial terminology means different things to different people. To reach a real understanding of the ancestral background of a patient or a research participant, workers need to move beyond simple "race" declarations. Such a declaration might unlock the door to a line of medical thinking, but it should be the opening to dialogue about ancestry and not the end of it. As noted by Mukhopadhyay and Moses (1997), the old racial categories mask the "very processes" that need to be understood. Designations that are ethnic-group specific may be more insightful than simple race classification.

Summary

Health workers need to be cognizant of the diverse history of race concepts, especially in the variability in interpretation of much of the racial terminology. Wherever possible, workers should move beyond simple race classification into the potentially more useful designations of ethnicity and detailed ancestral origins for the maximum impact of their important work.

References

American Anthropological Association. AAA statement on "race." *Anthropol Newsletter.* 1998;39(6):3.

Baker LD. Over a cliff into a brick wall. *Anthropol Newsletter.* 1998;39(1):16-17.

Barnouw V. *Physical anthropology and archaeology.* Chicago: The Dorsey Press; 1989.

Boyd WC. *Genetics and the races of man.* Boston: Little, Brown and Company; 1956.

Brace CL. Biocultural interaction and the mechanism of mosaic evolution in the emergence of "modern" morphology. *Am Anthropol.* 1995a;97(4):711-721.

Brace CL. Region does not mean "race"—reality versus convention in forensic anthropology. *J Forensic Sci.* 1995b;40(2):171-175.

Brace CL, Tracer DP, Yaroch LA, Robb J, Brandt K, Nelson AR. Clines and clusters versus "race": A test in ancient Egypt and the case of a death on the Nile. *Am J Phys Anthropol.* 1993; 36:1–31.

Brøberg G. Linnaeus' anthropology. In: Spencer F, ed. *History of physical anthropology: An encyclopedia.* New York: Garland Publishing Inc.; 1997:616-618.

Burris BG, Harris EF. Identification of race and sex from palate dimensions. *J Forensic Sci.* 1998;43(5):959-963.

Byers SN, Churchill SE, Curran B. Identification of Euro-Americans, Afro-Americans, and Amerindians from palatal dimensions. *J Forensic Sci.* 1997;42(1):3–9.

Cartmill M. The status of race concept in physical anthropology. *Am Anthropol.* 1999;100(3):651-660.

Coon CS. *The origin of races.* New York: Knopf; 1962.

Coon CS. *The living races of man.* New York: Knopf; 1965.

Craig E. Intercondylar shelf angle: A new method to determine race from the distal femur. *J Forensic Sci.* 1995;40(5):777-782.

Damon A. Race, ethnic group, and disease. In: Osborne RH, ed. *The biological and social meaning of race.* San Francisco: W.H. Freeman and Company; 1971:57-74.

Dobzhansky T. Race equality. In: Osborne RH, ed. *The biological and social meaning of race.* San Francisco: W.H. Freeman and Company; 1971:13-24.

Garn SM. *Human races.* Springfield, Ill: Charles C Thomas; 1962.

Gill GW. Challenge on the Frontier: Discerning American Indians from Whites osteologically. *J Forensic Sci.* 1995;40(5):783-788.

Gill, GW. The beauty of race and races. *Anthropol Newsletter.* 1998;39(3):1;4–5.

Gill GW, Rhine S, eds. *Skeletal attribution of race*. Maxwell Museum of Anthropology Anthropological Papers No 4; 1990.

Gregory S, Sanjek R, eds. *Race*. New Brunswick, N.J.: Rutgers University Press; 1994.

Harrison FV. Introduction: Expanding the discourse on "race." *Am Anthropol*. 1998;100(3):609-631.

Howells WW. The meaning of race. In: Osborne RH, ed. *The biological and social meaning of race*. San Francisco: W.H. Freeman and Company; 1971:3-10.

Keita SOY, Kittles RA. The persistence of racial thinking and the myth of racial divergence. *Am Anthropol*. 1997;99(3):534-544.

Kelso AJ. *Physical anthropology*. Philadelphia: J.B. Lippincott Company; 1974.

Kennedy KAR. But Professor, why teach race identification if races don't exist? *J Forensic Sci*. 1995;40(5):797–800.

King, JC. *The biology of race*. New York: Harcourt Brace Jovanovich Inc.; 1971.

Krantz GS. *Climatic races and descent groups*. North Quincy, Mass.: Christopher Publishing House; 1980.

Lasker GW. *Physical anthropology*. New York: Holt, Rinehart, and Winston; 1976.

Lieberman L. Gender and the deconstruction of the race concept. *Am Anthropol*. 1997;99(3):545-558.

Mellars P, Stringer C, eds. *The human revolution*. Princeton, N.J.: Princeton University Press; 1989.

Montagu A. The concept of race. In: Montagu A, ed. *The concept of race*. Westport, Conn.: Greenwood Press; 1964:12-28.

Montagu MFA. *Man's most dangerous myth: The fallacy of race*. New York: Columbia University Press; 1942.

Mukhopadhyay CC, Moses YT. Reestablishing "race" in anthropological discourse. *Am Anthropol*. 1997;99(3):517-533.

Osborne RH, ed. *The biological and social meaning of race*. San Francisco: W.H. Freeman and Company; 1971.

Ousley SD, Jantz RL. FORDISC 2.0: Personal computer forensic discriminant functions. Knoxville, Tenn.: The University of Tennessee; 1996.

Overfield T. *Biologic variation in health and illness: Race, age, and sex differences*. 2nd ed. Boca Raton, Fla.: CRC Press; 1995.

Paredes JA. Race is not something you can see. *Anthropol Newsletter*. 1997;38(9):1,6.

Relethford J. *The human species*. Mountain View, Calif.: Mayfield Publishing Company; 1990.

Sauer NJ. Forensic anthropology and the concept of race: If races don't exist, why are forensic anthropologists so good at identifying them? *Soc Sci Med*. 1992;34(2):107-111.

Sauer NJ. Applied anthropology and the concept of race: A legacy of Linneaus. National Association for the Practice of Anthropology, *Bulletin*. 1993;13:79-84.

Smedley A. "Race" and the construction of human identity. *Am Anthropol*. 1999; 100(3):690–702.

Spencer, F. Germany. In: Spencer F, ed. *History of physical anthropology: An encyclopedia*. New York: Garland Publishing Inc.; 1997:423-34.

Stewart TD. Review of "Man's most dangerous myth: The fallacy of race," by Montagu MFA, "Race: Science and politics," by Benedict R, "The races of mankind," by Benedict R and Weltfish G, and "Race, reason, and rubbish," by Dahlberg G. *Am J Physical Anthropol*. 1944; 2(3):321-322.

Stewart TD. *Essentials of forensic anthropology*. Springfield, Ill.: Charles C Thomas; 1979.

Stewart TD, Newman MT. An historical résumé of the concept of differences in Indian types. *Am Anthropol*. 1951;53:19–36.

Studstill JD. Race, ethnicity and baby's bathwater. *Anthropol Newsletter*. 1998;39(1):16-17.

Templeton AR. Human races: A genetic and evolutionary perspective. *Am Anthropol*. 1999;100(3):632–650.

Ubelaker DH. Skeletons testify: Anthropology in forensic science, AAPA Luncheon Address: April 12, 1996. *Yearbook Phys Anthropol*. 1996; 39:229-244.

Visweswaran K. Race and the culture of anthropology. *Am Anthropol*. 1998;100(1):70-83.

Webster's new international dictionary of the English language. 2nd ed. Springfield, Mass.: G. & C. Merriam Company; 1941.

Wolpoff M, Caspari R. *Race and human evolution*. New York: Simon & Schuster; 1997.

Chapter 3

ETHICAL ISSUES *and* UNETHICAL CONDUCT:

Race, Racism, and the Abuse of Human Subjects in Research

Elizabeth Heitman, PhD, and Alan L. Wells, MPH

It is an irony of ethical development that theoretical insight and practical reform result more often from scandal and catastrophe than from thoughtful consideration of moral ideals in less turbulent times. As repeatedly documented by scholars of the history and ethics of medicine, medical research offers a classic example of this phenomenon: Authoritative ethical standards for research with human subjects have typically been developed in response to the inhumane and abusive actions of researchers. Starting with the atrocities committed by German physicians in the wartime pursuit of the Nazi medical agenda and continuing into the more subtle consequences of contemporary genetic research, the identification of ethical issues, the refinement and expansion of ethical standards, and the establishment of specific regulations governing human research have continued to come predominantly in response to research activities that put vulnerable individuals and groups at risk of harm.

The history of medical research offers a powerful illustration of how ethical reflection lags behind practice and technological developments, and how grossly unethical conduct may occur in the gap. This history also documents how science and medicine are influenced by the prejudices of the society in which they operate, and how their ethical underpinnings may be flawed by society's ills. Increasingly, contemporary analysis of the history of modern medical research demonstrates that while research subjects have indeed suffered harms as a result of investigators' unrestrained zeal, many of the worst abuses have been committed against persons whose rights and intrinsic humanity were denied by the society in which the researchers operated.

This chapter addresses the role of race and racism in the ethics of research with human subjects, and the ethical issues raised by researchers' race-based considerations. After a brief overview of the historical development of modern medical research and its early ethical norms, the chapter explores how concepts of race affected the ethical standards applied to medical research in three cases of egregiously unethical conduct: the Nazi research of the 1930s and 1940s, the Japanese biological warfare research of the same period, and the 1932–1972 U.S. Public Health Service (PHS) syphilis study at Tuskegee, Alabama. These cases illustrate how racism can pervade the practice of medical experimentation and biomedical science even when researchers and governmental authorities acknowledge the need to protect subjects from the potential harms of research.

The chapter then considers two areas of current biomedical research in which race raises ethical issues not fully resolved in history: the development of effective pharmacotherapy for the prevention and treatment of HIV/AIDS in developing countries, and the Human Genome Diversity Project, an international effort to map the genetic variability of some 4000–8000 specific human groups. In both these endeavors, conflicting definitions of the research in question and researchers' attempts to tailor the work to the needs and cultural values of potential subjects have created debate about the universal applicability of ethical principles and the protections required in western democracies.

The cases of unethical and ethically ambiguous research examined here illustrate that the broader social context in which research is conducted inherently shapes the framing of the question and the goals that research is meant to serve. They also depict how even research into the nature and significance of health-related differences between groups is at risk of incorporating racist views of difference. Moreover, they highlight how regulation alone may be unable to prevent racism's subtler effects on biomedical science, as their contextual causes are often visible only in retrospect, and thus are not easily amenable to a policy response.

The Rise of Experimental Medicine and Early Reflection on the Ethics of Research with Human Subjects

The practice and ethical standards of medical research as they are known today are little more than a few decades old. The medical sciences from which modern research developed—microscopy and microscopic anatomy, pathology, bacteriology, biochemistry, and physiology—date from only the early 1800s. Their pioneers worked predominantly in the medical universities of Germany and Austria, where the developing theories and techniques of laboratory medicine were increasingly applied to surgery and therapeutics in the late 1800s (Bordley and Harvey 1976; Nuland 1988). Elsewhere, few physicians had any exposure to laboratory medicine or the principles of experimentation before the 1900s. During this period, the small percentage of U.S. physicians interested in specialty practice, and wealthy enough to travel abroad, sought training in Europe. They returned with the skills to engage in rudimentary laboratory diagnosis and small-scale empiric evaluation of medications.

Scientific medicine and organized clinical research took root in the United States in 1893 with the opening of Johns Hopkins University Medical School, whose founding faculty had been rigorously trained in Germany (Bordley and Harvey 1976).

However, few medical schools adopted the Hopkins model until after the Carnegie Foundation's 1910 Flexner Report, which advocated restructuring medical schools in line with the Hopkins approach. Abraham Flexner was subsequently engaged by John D. Rockefeller, Jr., to distribute $50 million to medical schools able and willing to undertake the transformation. By the 1920s the scope and amount of medical research had increased tremendously (Bordley and Harvey 1976; Nuland 1988).

Nonetheless, before the 1930s, research in even these medical schools was little more than what medical historian David Rothman has called a "cottage industry" (Rothman 1991, p. 18). Most studies combined patient care with laboratory techniques and an experimental approach to the development of new therapies. Typically the subject and researcher had an established doctor–patient relationship, and both parties viewed experimental procedures as being in the patient's interest. Early on, many physician researchers were aware of the potential conflict between the well-being of the patient-subject and the demands of science and were careful to articulate the physician's duty to safeguard the patient's welfare. In 1865, French surgeon and physiologist Claude Bernard wrote in *An Introduction to Experimental Medicine* that "The principle of medical and surgical morality. . . consists in never performing on a man an experiment which might be harmful to him to any extent, even though the result might be highly advantageous to science, i.e., to the health of others" (Bernard in Reiser et al. 1978).

Other physician-researchers readily identified the vulnerability of certain groups of patients, and advocated for the physician's duty both to protect patient-subjects and to ensure patients' willingness to participate in medical experiments. In the United States, physician Charles Francis Withington expressed concern in 1886 that "(i)n the older countries of Europe especially, where the life and happiness of the so-called lower classes are perhaps held more cheaply than with us, enthusiastic devotees of science are very apt to encroach upon the rights of the patient in ways which cannot be justified" (Withington in Reiser et al. 1978). Withington insisted that patients have "a right to immunity from experiments merely as such, and outside of therapeutic application" (Withington in Reiser et al. 1978). Moreover, he maintained that physician researchers should always seek the patient's permission, and should call for volunteers for experiments with no medical benefit. In Germany, the Prussian Minister for Spiritual etc. Affairs (sic) laid down essentially these same guidelines in a 1901 directive to the heads of a variety of clinics and hospitals (Howard-Jones 1982). Generally, the philosophy espoused by Withington was the professional ideal for medical research in North America and Europe into the 1930s (Rothman 1991).

By the late 1920s, many U.S. medical schools and their affiliated hospitals had recognized the advantages that research offered. As the number of researchers grew, the cottage industry became more institutionalized and researchers became more interested in the benefits that their work could provide to society. There was a growing sense that all physicians should engage in research at some level, and patients typically believed that they had a certain obligation to society and to their physicians to take part in research when offered experimental therapy (Schwitalla 1929 in Reiser et al. 1978).

Nonetheless, as early as Walter Reed's yellow fever studies in the 1890s, the public expressed outrage when nontherapeutic research was shown to cause harm (Rothman 1991). By the 1920s, growing interest in larger-scale research more frequently led to nontherapeutic studies with unconsenting subjects in orphanages, asylums, and public hospitals, yet such studies typically prompted vigorous public criticism when exposed. In New York, research into a diagnostic test for syphilis conducted on several hundred children led to calls for legal sanctions against doctors who conducted nontherapeutic studies on anyone without consent (Lederer 1985).

In Germany, press coverage and public criticism of nontherapeutic investigations resulted in governmental hearings in 1930. In 1931, the German Ministry of the Interior issued guidelines for human experimentation that emphasized the therapeutic goals of research; the need for subjects' consent based on full disclosure; the protection of minors and persons affected by social deprivation; and documentation of the experimental treatment and the subject's consent (Howard-Jones 1982). While these guidelines were not legally binding, they provide a clear indication of professional research ethics and related tensions in research in Germany before Hitler came to power.

The consideration of modern research ethics typically begins with the aftermath of World War II and the revelation of research atrocities committed by Nazi physicians. The war provided the impetus for the exponential growth of medical research internationally and accelerated the shift from patient-oriented experimentation to knowledge-oriented research that had begun in the 1920s. The rapid expansion and institutionalization of research led to the phenomenal advances for which medical science is now known, as well as to its most significant ethical controversies. Both Axis and Allied governments approached research as a facet of military and political strategy, but the racist political agendas of Nazi Germany and Japan corrupted both the ethics and the science behind their work. Wartime research had horrific consequences for countless men, women, and children involuntarily subjected to research that cast "non-Aryans" and non-Japanese as subhuman beings undeserving of ethical concern.

Research, Race, and Ethics in the World War II Era

Nazi Racism, Medicine, and Public Health

Between the first and second world wars, Germany's scientific and medical establishment went from being the world's undisputed leader in medical research to being the system best known for the perversion of science and the flagrant misapplication of medicine under the Nazi regime. Prior to Hitler's rise to power, German medical ethical standards were not only consistent with those of physicians in other western democracies, German physicians' public debate on the ethics of research reflected considerable insight into the ethical conflicts that research physicians still face today. Under Hitler, German doctors—and the medical enterprise as a whole—were transformed by the racism of the Nazi party, which subverted the ethics of medicine and science with previously discredited anthropological theories of race.

The origins of Nazi racism lay in the national myth of a germanic Volk, an archetypal people that German anthropologists attempted to document in the mid-1800s with the tools of the developing sciences of pathology and genealogy-based genetics. By the late 1800s, the epidemiological and archeological research of German pathologist Rudolf Virchow had all but discredited the pseudo-science behind German claims of racially pure ancestry (Nuland 1988), but Germany's devastation after World War I fostered a resurgence of the myth of racial purity (Weiss 1996). In *Mein Kampf*, Hitler reasserted the theory of the biological superiority of the "true" German people, whom he identified as "Aryan."* He defined the Nazi's divine mission as that of "assembling and preserving the most valuable stocks of basic racial elements in this people...[and] raising them to a dominant position" (Lifton 1986, p. 17). Robert Lifton, who chronicled the Nazi medical research agenda in *The Nazi Doctors: Medical Killing and the Psychology of Genocide*, suggests that the Nazis saw the state as a "biocracy," a system of rule by divine prerogative conferred by the biology of race (Lifton 1986).

The Nazis systematically took over and reorganized the entire medical profession in Germany under the process known as "synchronization" or Gleichschaltung (Lifton 1986, p. 33). Physicians were indoctrinated with the theory that racial purity was an essential medical goal, and that all "non-Aryan" peoples were a potential threat to the health of the German nation. Jews in particular were cast as subhuman, and were identified as the "primary matter of everything negative" (Goldhagen 1997, p. 412). The Nazis' "scientific racism" advocated a biomedical cure for the nation's ills, which began with the sterilization of "non-Aryans" and weaker populations, such as the physically and mentally handicapped and the mentally ill, and ended with "euthanasia"—the direct medical killing of "useless mouths," persons with "lives not worth living" (Lifton 1986; Goldhagen 1997; Ivy 1947 in Reiser et al. 1978).

Surprisingly, many historians overlook the Nazis' use of the language and methods of public health to promote "scientific racism" and race-based medical killing. Under the auspices of racial hygiene, the Nazis developed strong epidemiological surveillance programs and population health campaigns, years before other western countries adopted similar approaches to disease prevention. As Robert Proctor documents in *The Nazi War on Cancer* (Proctor 1999), the Nazis made a clear distinction between "negative" and "positive" racial hygiene. "Positive" efforts sought to promote the breeding of a "superior" population; "negative" efforts were designed to reduce the number of "unfit" persons in society and to limit their reproduction. While extensive public health campaigns against smoking, drinking, and environmental pollution were intended to protect the supposedly superior genetic materials of the

---

* "Aryan" refers loosely to several seminomadic tribal groups ranging from Poland to Central Asia who entered India through an uneven series of southwestern migrations between 2000 and 3000 BCE. Their cultural practices influenced Hinduism through socioreligious narratives known as the Vedas. In the mid-1800s, German linguists documented the similarities between Vedic Sanskrit and classic Germanic languages, and several anthropologists sought to link the Germans to these ancient peoples. The Nazis used the term Aryan, incorrectly, to refer to a pure German race, and adopted Vedic symbols for purity—most notably the swastika (Sanskrit for "good health" or "long life")— for political purposes.

"true" German stock, public health claims were also made for the benefits of eliminating the weaker and diseased elements of society.

Screening for disease played an essential role in public health activities aimed at racial hygiene, as Germany became "obsessed with tracking, diagnosing, registering, grading, and selecting" its citizens (Proctor 1999, p. 40). Proctor describes the Nazi period as "an era of mass screenings." Nazi epidemiologists drew up extensive catalogues and maps detailing the geographic distribution of race and genetic diseases. Screening was a particularly important component of the war on cancer, an effort central to the Nazi medical agenda. Cancer and malignancy were also common Nazi metaphors for undesirable persons and activities—the Jewish people in particular were often portrayed as a cancer in the body of the German nation, and individual Jews often referred to as tumors. By cloaking racism in the rhetoric of public health, the Nazis were able to portray the imprisonment and medical killing of Jews and other so-called unworthy persons as part of a global campaign to eliminate health threats and promote the health of a racially pure Germany (Proctor 1999).

Much of the healing–killing paradox of Nazi medicine unfolded in a network of internment centers where physicians' acquiescence to the ideology of racial cure undermined their professional ethics of research. The model concentration camp was established at Dachau almost immediately after the Nazis came to power. The camp at Auschwitz became especially committed to research and the medicalized killing of Jews. Lifton contends that the essential word in the equation of healing and killing was Sonderbehandlung, or "special treatment." The term not only detoxified killing and facilitated its routine acceptance, it simultaneously "infused that killing with a near-mystical priority" for the Auschwitz physician as a necessary, medically appropriate intervention (Lifton 1986, p. 150).

Lifton suggests that the Nazis' medical experiments fell into two categories: those sponsored by the regime for a specific military or ideological purpose and those done out of alleged individual scientific interest by more enterprising SS physicians. Party-sanctioned research efforts typically were informed by the ideology of racial and genetic purity, the most egregious examples of which included sterilization and reproductive experiments, the various experiments of the "Hygienic Institute" at Auschwitz's "Block 10," and the macabre collection of corpses at the "anthropological museum" at Auschwitz. These experiments are documented extensively in Nuremberg Trial records and a wide variety of Holocaust studies. In its essence, the research was conducted with no regard for the value of human life or subjects' pain or suffering, and lacked even basic scientific merit (Ivy 1947 in Reiser et al. 1978).

The crossover between medical research and euthanasia is well illustrated by the activities of the Hygienic Institute and the anthropological museum. The culture medium used in experiments at the Hygienic Institute was readily obtained from huge quantities of human tissue excised from the bodies of prisoners executed at Auschwitz (Lifton 1986, p. 289). Hundreds of people were executed in order that researchers at the anthropology museum could preserve their skulls and other body parts as specimens (Ivy 1947 in Reiser et al. 1978). In a memo requesting the skulls of executed Russian Jews, SS Captain Dr. August Hirt reported that the goal of this collection was to "acquire tangible scientific research material" that would "represent… a repulsive but typical species of sub-humanity" (Lifton 1986, p. 285).

Block 10's sterilization experiments were notorious for mutilating relatively healthy young Jewish men and women in order to investigate the potential of radiation and surgical techniques for the sterilization of "non-Aryans." Surgical investigations of the effects of X-rays on the reproductive organs of both men and women were often fatal. Most died of their wounds, and survivors were often executed. Researchers contended that their subjects were "guinea pigs" whose "deaths mattered little" (Lifton 1986, p. 283).

Auschwitz was open to virtually any medical use of human subjects, including clinical trials for commercial interests and surgical training (Lifton 1986; Ivy 1947 in Reiser et al. 1978). SS Captain Dr. Helmuth Vetter organized pharmaceutical trials with prisoners for the Bayer Group (Lifton 1986). German medical students used Auschwitz facilities as a surgical laboratory, and trainees routinely removed or surgically manipulated the limbs and organs of Jewish prisoners with the reassurance that their educational efforts were not harmful because the prisoners were condemned to death whatever the outcome of surgery.

Dr. Johann Paul Kremer, anatomy professor from the University of Münster, was one of the only university professors to serve as an SS camp doctor. Lifton documents that Kremer's interest in starvation led him to seek out "proper specimens" at Auschwitz, typically debilitated prisoners slated for death. When he was ready to do a dissection, he took a history focused on weight loss, then had an SS orderly inject phenol directly into the person's heart. Immediately upon the subject's death, Kremer and his assistant removed segments of the liver, spleen, and pancreas (Lifton 1986, p. 292). Occasionally Kremer examined or photographed his subjects prior to killing and dissecting them.

Certainly the most infamous medical personality to work at Auschwitz was Dr. Josef Mengele, whose extensive research on identical twins, most of whom were children, was examined at length in testimony to the War Tribunal in Nuremberg. To many, Mengele was the ultimate Nazi doctor, whose work embodied the research process at Auschwitz. Mengele's graduate medical work focused on the study of genealogy and genetic abnormalities. He arrived at Auschwitz with a research agenda based on finding identical twins to study hereditary traits and "relations between disease, racial types, and miscegenation" (Lifton 1986, p. 348). There he routinely conducted extensive measurements on Jewish twins, then injected their hearts with phenol in order to dissect them for further study or the collection of specimens. Mengele was known as a manic collector of things human, including dwarf corpses, gallstones, and eyes. His fascination with eyes led to the infamous experiments in which he injected various substances into the eyes of brown-eyed Jewish children in an attempt to make them "Nordic" (blue). In his tenure at Auschwitz, Mengele killed an unknown number of children under the auspices of research (Lifton 1986, p. 343).

When the Allied forces liberated the concentration camps at the end of the war, they were horrified to discover the camps' research facilities and the state of the prisoners who were research subjects. The subsequent military tribunals that investigated and tried Nazi physicians for war crimes and crimes against humanity found that their experiments were "the product of coordinated policy-making and planning at high governmental, military, and Nazi Party levels, conducted as a part of the total war effort" (The Nuremberg Code in Reiser et al. 1978). Although the vast majority of Nazi physician researchers and their assistants escaped prosecution for their part in the medicalized killing of Jews (Weiss 1996), the investigation of Nazi medical research by military prosecutors, and the later conviction of 16 physician researchers, was reported internationally.* The documented horror of the Nazi medical campaign prompted the Nuremberg Tribunal to articulate ethical standards by which the researchers could be judged. The Nuremberg Code, which turned on the concept that "the voluntary consent of the human subject is absolutely essential," articulated an international standard that became the bedrock of modern research ethics (The Nuremberg Code in Reiser et al. 1978).

However, even as the Nuremberg Tribunal sentenced Nazi researchers to death for crimes against humanity, U.S. investigators and the International Military Tribunal for the Far East, known as the Tokyo Tribunal, uncovered overwhelming evidence that Japanese researchers in the Pacific war theater had conducted medical research that also qualified as crimes against humanity. Investigators documented extensive lethal medical experimentation conducted by Japanese physicians on Allied prisoners and the ethnic Chinese population of occupied Manchuria, particularly related to the development of biological weapons. In sharp contrast to the relative openness of the trial, imprisonment, and execution of Nazi doctors, many of the Tokyo Tribunal's findings related to the Japanese research agenda and its abuses were quickly classified as information vital to U.S. security and kept secret (Dower 1999; Harris 1994; Endicott and Hagerman 1998). Until the 1980s, the history of Japanese medical researchers' abuses of human subjects during World War II was almost wholly unknown in the West (Girdwood 1985). What is now known about Japanese wartime research clearly documents more than a decade of atrocities motivated by racist ideology, and a subsequent cover-up of biological warfare research in which political interests took precedence over justice.

Research and Racism in Japanese Camps in Manchuria

Since 1980, a number of scholarly works based on personal interviews and U.S. and Japanese government documents have confirmed what were once only rumors that Japanese research in occupied Manchuria was comparable to the worst atrocities of Nazi Germany (Dower 1999; Harris 1994; Endicott and Hagerman 1998; Powell 1980; Powell 1981; Gold 1996). Much like their German counterparts, in the early 1930s technically expert Japanese medical researchers were corrupted by racist ideology to support militaristic governmental policies based on an age-old Japanese con-

---

* Six of the 46 physicians tried by the Nuremberg Military Tribunal in 1947 for medical war crimes and crimes against humanity were executed; the rest were imprisoned for varying periods of time. However, the German courts responsible for trying many accused of taking part in medical experimentation and euthanasia typically absolved them for "following orders." Josef Mengele fled Germany to avoid criminal prosecution by the Americans, and lived out his life under an assumed identity in exile (Weiss 1996).

cept of racial superiority. Throughout the war, Japanese medical investigators were responsible for the deaths of countless people subjected to hideous medical research in support of Japan's racist military goals.

As a result of Japan's physical and subsequent cultural isolation, the Japanese had long been ethnocentric. As historian Sheldon Harris describes in *Factories of Death: Japanese Biological Warfare, 1932–1945, and the American Cover-Up*, the Japanese believed that they were a special race of people whose "pure" racial stock and unique culture were superior to all others (Harris 1994, pp. 44–45). This superiority implied their destiny to rule over the other purportedly inferior peoples of Asia, a destiny the Japanese military sought to fulfill in the 1930s with the invasion of China and the Pacific islands. Japanese medical research was closely aligned with these military goals, as many people believed that biological and chemical warfare were essential to Japan's wartime success.

The invasion of China provided a perfect experimental population for the testing of Japan's biological and chemical weapons. Japanese medical scientists turned Manchuria into a biological and chemical laboratory for weapons research from the moment that Japan occupied the region (1931–1932) until its surrender in August of 1945 (Harris 1994; Endicott and Hagerman 1998). Japanese research facilities were scattered throughout Manchuria. The largest of these camps, Ping Fan, was disguised as a lumber mill, and rail cars transporting hundreds of Chinese peasants to die as research subjects were often topped with a row of lumber to avoid the suspicion of onlookers. Japanese doctors and medical students who worked in these facilities later commented that they typically referred to their subjects as maruta or "logs," reinforcing the perception that the Chinese were subhuman experimental material (Harris 1994, p. 39; Girdwood 1985). The Chinese were not the only "subhuman" racial group to be subjected to medical research: to test the hypothesis that Anglo-Saxons responded differently from other groups to illness, Japanese physicians used Allied prisoners of war for a number of experiments (Harris 1994; Girdwood 1985). Published reports of the findings of research done in the camps typically referred to experiments with "Manchurian monkeys" rather than human subjects. However, in Japanese medical society, the reality of human experimentation was an open secret (Harris 1994, p. 63).

The biggest hub for chemical and biological warfare research was at Harbin, in the far northeastern side of the province. Here the notorious Ping Fan center, also known as Unit 731, was run by Major Dr. Ishii Shiro, a military physician trained in microbiology who was instrumental in persuading the Japanese government that biological weapons were the key to winning the war (Harris 1994; Gold 1996). Unit 731 was the Japanese equivalent to the medical killing complex at Auschwitz, but the death toll from Ishii's work was unrivaled by that of any of his Nazi contemporaries. Experimenters attempted to cover every conceivable aspect of spreading and preventing disease, including the design and testing of bomb casings intended to maximize the dispersion of pathogens. Different strains and dosages of specific germs were tested in camps for their ability to kill, and the most lethal were subsequently field tested on segments of the Chinese population (Harris 1994, pp. 60–61).

Field experiments and epidemiological tracking were crucial to the Japanese development of biological weapons. Entire villages were killed in the effort to determine that typhoid germs placed in public water wells would lead to widespread infection; and such field experiments often involved large-scale official deception of Chinese community leaders. Harris describes how, at the Unit 100 camp in Changchun, Japanese researchers intentionally caused a cholera outbreak. Ishii approached local authorities to announce that cholera was moving throughout their community, and that the general population had to be inoculated. The authorities consented; however the "vaccine" was actually a solution containing live cholera. The inoculation stations also offered cholera-laced food and drink. Similarly, at Nanking epidemics were spread with "special gifts" of holiday foods, such as dumplings and candies, injected with typhoid, anthrax, or paratyphoid (Harris 1994, p. 77). Japanese researchers carefully documented the extent and severity of the spread of disease during these tests, obtaining epidemiological data for biological weapons design.

The development and manufacture of vaccines against biological weapons was also a vital part of Japanese physicians' work in the Manchurian camps. Harris reports that at least 20 million doses of vaccine were prepared each year of operation at Unit 731, and untold millions more were produced at camp centers in Changchun and Nanking (Harris 1994). The operations at Unit 731 involved special teams who produced the vaccines, technicians who tested them on human subjects, and pathologists who recorded subjects' physiological reactions, usually on the dying or the newly dead.

Like its counterpart in Germany, the Japanese wartime government reorganized medical practice and re-educated physicians consistent with its nationalist goals. Many physicians and medical trainees were sent to Manchuria as a part of the overall biological and chemical weapons research effort, where they dissected research subjects to evaluate the effects of particular experimental interventions. Chinese research subjects were also used for trainees' surgery practice, including dissections with and without anesthesia, hypodermic injection practice, and the recovery of tissue specimens for commercial use (Gold 1996). Japanese civil servants frequently worked with physicians and technicians in the military-medical complexes in Manchuria. As one civilian employee of Unit 731 later testified, "I did not want to experiment on maruta. The major reason a lot of people joined was to protect health with hygiene, and the pay was good" (Gold 1996, p. 217).

As in Germany, the nature and scope of Japanese medical research was unknown to the Allied forces before the end of the war, although the FBI and other U.S. intelligence agencies had been concerned about the possibility of Japanese biological weapons research in China as early as 1941 (Harris 1994). When Japan surrendered in 1945, Ishii evacuated his personnel and fellow scientists from the Manchurian research facilities to Japan, and attempted to destroy the camps. Members of the U.S. intelligence community soon learned that Japanese military physicians had engaged in biological warfare research, and that Ishii had been the lead investigator. Because Manchuria was one of the territories occupied by the Soviet Union, the U.S. government was particularly concerned that biological warfare information not fall into the hands of the Soviet army (Dower 1999), which captured, tried, and executed remaining Manchurian research camp personnel as war criminals. U.S. officials sought to track Ishii and his colleagues to interrogate them as quickly as possible (Harris 1994).

The Tokyo Tribunal's legal teams introduced a post-Nuremberg assessment of war crimes in which abusive medical experimentation was included in Class C, "crimes against humanity" (Dower 1999). While prosecutors with the Tokyo Tribunal learned that Japanese research practices paralleled the horrors of Nazi medical experimentation, Japanese medical research in Manchuria was never publicly investigated and researchers were never put on trial. Many serious charges were dismissed in the effort to bargain for biological warfare data thought to be essential to U.S. security interests. Ishii and the officers and researchers of Unit 731 were granted "blanket secret immunity" (Dower 1999) because, as summarized in a memo entitled "Intelligence Information on Bacteriological Warfare from 1947," if they were tried, it would be impossible for the United States to keep vital Japanese biological warfare information secret (Harris 1994). The dismissal of charges was also facilitated by the Tokyo Tribunal's inability to find a clear Japanese governmental counterpoint to the Nazi medical agenda that advocated genocide (Dower 1999), despite the larger death toll from the Manchurian germ warfare research.

Historian John W. Dower has concluded that the Tokyo Tribunal's response to the Japanese medical war crimes was largely the result of the Allied forces' fear of communism, the sudden onset of the cold war, and the increasing public ennui with the length and complexity of the proceedings themselves (Dower 1999). However, Chinese critics of the proceedings make a persuasive argument that U.S. war crimes investigators were able to disregard the victims of Japanese biological weapons research knowing that the American public would not identify with the unfamiliar Manchurian Chinese in even the limited way that they had with the European Jews.*

The U.S. government ultimately appropriated a considerable amount of Japanese research data for its own purposes (Harris 1994; Endicott and Hagerman 1998). Documentation from U.S. military officials involved with Japanese researchers indicated that they deliberately sought to recover biological weapons data in order to take advantage of work that they knew could never be repeated. U.S. authorities acknowledged that similar data "could not be obtained in our own laboratories because of scruples attached to human experimentation" (Harris 1994, p. 66). Moreover, the Japanese research had been carried out at a cost of many millions of dollars and years of work that the United States could not afford to replicate.

Had the proceedings and findings of the Tokyo Tribunal been publicized, the U.S. military's decision to incorporate Japanese biological weapons data into its own germ warfare experimentation likely would have been controversial among U.S. medical scientists. As early as the 1930s, many investigators had already questioned whether it was ever ethical to use the findings of research conducted in violation of basic principles of informed consent (Rothman 1991; Howard-Jones 1982). This debate

---

* Internet sites dedicated to publicizing the horrors of Japanese wartime activities in Manchuria condemn the United States for anti-Chinese racism. Search particularly under the term "Unit 731."

continued after the war regarding the legitimacy of using Nazi data gathered from torturous studies on Jewish prisoners (Moe 1984). Chinese critics maintain that the U.S. military's granting of immunity to Ishii and his colleagues and the subsequent use of their work* were crimes no different from the original research that caused the suffering and deaths of millions of people. Moreover, they claim that the U.S. government's silence about these events and the continuing public ignorance in the United States since their disclosure are further evidence of westerners' ongoing racist disregard for the Manchurians, subjugating human rights concerns to strategic military interests.

Medical Research Abuse in the United States and the Race-Based Tuskegee Syphilis Trial

To the 21st-century reader, the eloquence of the Nuremberg Code and the classification of research abuse as a war crime suggest that ethical standards for informed consent were uniform for U.S. researchers of the 1940s. However, consent practices were highly variable, and the growth of research as an institutional activity often left the United States research community open to criticism. During the Nuremberg proceedings, Nazi doctors attempted to defend their work by citing U.S. research in which prisoners and other captive populations were intentionally infected or otherwise harmed in order for researchers to study the pathology and progression of a specific condition (Hornblum 1998).

The Tribunal did not accept the Nazis' claim that some U.S. research practices paralleled their own. It is undeniable, however, that both before and after the war medical researchers in the United States often did not adhere to the Nuremberg Code's high standards of free and voluntary consent for research subjects. Even after the World Medical Association published international standards of research ethics in the 1964 Declaration of Helsinki (World Medical Association 2000), the need for subjects' consent was not universally respected by U.S. medical investigators, and the 1960s saw much debate about the meaning of consent in research. In 1966, amid the controversy, the U.S. Surgeon General issued guidelines for the institutional review of Public Health Service (PHS)-funded research that included provisions for protecting the rights and welfare of research subjects, obtaining subjects' informed consent, and assessing the risks and potential medical benefits to subjects of the research (U.S. Public Health Service 1966).

As if to underscore the need for formal ethical oversight, later that same year Harvard anesthesiologist Henry K. Beecher assailed U.S. researchers' failure to seek subjects' consent in a highly controversial review of 100 studies published "in an excellent journal" in 1964 (Beecher 1966). His essay outlined 22 examples of unethical research practices, predominantly involving the involuntary enrollment of incompetent or extremely vulnerable subjects in risky, nontherapeutic studies. Beyond his

---

* Recent work by two Canadian analysts has suggested that the U.S. Army employed Japanese biological weapons researchers and conducted additional biological warfare research in Korea and China in the 1950s (Endicott and Hagerman 1998).

critique of the projects themselves, Beecher decried the lack of ethical concern among authorities at the institutions where they were conducted, and the medical professionals who allowed the studies to become part of the authoritative literature without objection.

Beecher's observations were echoed dramatically six years later in 1972, when Associated Press (AP) reporter Jean Heller rocked the medical community with an exposé of the U.S. Public Health Service's Tuskegee Syphilis Study, breaking the news that for 40 years PHS physicians had conducted research that denied effective treatment to a group of poor, uneducated African-American men with syphilis. The involvement of federal, state, and local health officials, the support of private medical foundations, and the fact that 13 reports from the project had been published in respected medical journals made the study's calculated deception of its subjects a scandal that evoked images of Nazi experimentation for many Americans (Jones 1993).

The history of the now infamous 40-year Study of Untreated Syphilis in the Negro Male in Macon County, Alabama, has been carefully detailed by ethicist James H. Jones in *Bad Blood: The Tuskegee Syphilis Experiment* (Jones 1993). The study had its origins in a PHS screening and treatment project that began in 1930 in six southern states. The project sought to determine how best to control syphilis in a variety of circumstances in the rural south. Initially, men who tested positive received treatment with mercury and two arsenic compounds called arsphenamine and neoarsphenamine. Although this regimen was the standard of care at that time, the men received a dose that would not cure them, but which doctors thought would leave them noninfectious (Jones 1993). Because they believed that the rural population would not fully understand the project or even recognize the term "syphilis," public health workers never fully described their goals or methods to the men they tested. Rather, they said that they were testing people for "bad blood," a phrase from the local vernacular that was deceptively general and had multiple meanings, and said little about the treatment provided. Few men refused the offer of testing, and some 1400 were treated during the 18 months that the program was funded.

When funding for the project was not renewed in the midst of the Depression, PHS physician Dr. Taliaferro Clark noted in his final report that the high prevalence of syphilis in Macon County offered an "unparalleled opportunity" to study the effects of the untreated disease (Jones 1993, p. 91). Clark was particularly interested in providing a Negro* counterpart to the Oslo Study of untreated syphilis, a retrospective study of Norwegian syphilis patients followed in an Oslo clinic from 1891 to 1919. In 1929, investigators from the Oslo study had reported that the cardiovascular effects of tertiary syphilis were considerable, while neurologic effects were rare. This finding contradicted the common medical assumption that White men were more affected by the neurologic effects of syphilis than the cardiovascular effects, which were presumed to affect Black men more significantly. Clark proposed that some of the work of the demonstration project could be salvaged by conducting a prospective

* The term and variable capitalization of Negro as used here reflects the language of the medical literature cited and the terminology used by PHS investigators at the time.

study on the effects of untreated syphilis among the residents of Macon County to establish the relative importance of cardiovascular versus neurologic effects in a Negro population.

The Tuskegee study was based on the hypothesis that the clinical course of syphilis was different for the two races. The theoretical framework for this hypothesis emerged in the United States in the early 1800s, as physicians attempted identify differences between the races, often as part of an attempted justification of slavery (Jones in Reich 1978). Even at the turn of the century many southern physicians contended that Negroes had different natural immunity and reactions to disease than Whites, and almost all diseases were understood on a Black–White clinical continuum that stressed the effects of individual predisposition and behavior. Sexuality was of special interest to advocates of racial medicine, who claimed that sexual promiscuity and physical weakness were intrinsic racial characteristics that explained the high incidence of syphilis among Negroes. As Jones observes, the availability of the data on untreated syphilis in a White cohort made a parallel study of the latent stage in Black men an appealing epidemiologic project to researchers, who contended that "syphilis in the negro is in many respects a different disease from syphilis in the White" (Jones 1993). They anticipated that their study would emphasize these differences.

At the end of 1932, Clark and PHS physician Dr. Raymond Vondelehr gathered the support of the state and county health officials, local physicians, and the Tuskegee Institute to conduct a six-month long study that would identify significant complications among men who tested positive and whose clinical history indicated late latent syphilis. All of the study subjects received treatment, although mercury and neoarsphenamine were not consistently available and the short-term regimen provided was known to be ineffective (Jones 1993, p. 118). Toward the end of the six months, Vondelehr proposed long-term surveillance of the group, with the ultimate goal of conducting autopsies to establish the final clinical outcome of the men's latent infection. Because the minimal treatment that the subjects had received was insufficient to reverse their infection, Vondelehr was confident that the original study group could be considered "untreated" if they receive no further effective intervention. By early 1934 he gradually organized local doctors, public health officials, and the Black leadership of the Tuskegee Institute in a secret agreement to deny effective treatment to 399 study subjects while the PHS regularly documented the progression of their conditions as compared with 200 controls.

Throughout the course of the study, researchers insisted that their surveillance was much like an experiment in nature. The poor Black farmers enrolled in the project were extremely unlikely to have sought treatment for their syphilis under normal circumstances and their almost certain inability to pay for care would have prevented them from receiving effective intervention had they sought help. When penicillin replaced heavy metal therapy as the standard of care for syphilis in 1947, researchers insisted that the availability of effective therapy made it even more essential to continue the study. The PHS engaged a sort of ethical inversion, claiming that the availability of penicillin made the study an opportunity that could never again be repeated, as it would be impossible to find another infected group so large

(Jones 1993, p. 181). Jones details how a comprehensive review of the study by PHS officials in 1951 ultimately focused not on the ethics of the denial of treatment, but on the extent to which the study had been contaminated by intervention, including antibiotics.

By 1951, PHS officials should have been familiar with the Nuremberg Tribunal and the provisions of the Code governing informed consent and the researcher's obligation to protect subjects from the risk of harm. The Tuskegee study violated both the spirit and the letter of the Nuremberg Code, but PHS researchers saw no similarity between Tuskegee and the Nazi experiments. Even the 1966 Surgeon General's mandate for the ethical review of research protocols had little effect on their view of the project. Jones concludes that the PHS officials responsible for oversight of research activities had been co-opted by their own familiarity with the Tuskegee study, and were unable to see their own complicity in unethical research (Jones 1993, p. 181).

It was a relative outsider who eventually brought an end to the Tuskegee study. Peter Buxton, a social worker at a PHS venereal disease clinic in San Francisco in the mid-1960s, was shocked to learn of the study, and became convinced by reading its published reports that the project was unethical. Between 1966 and 1968 Buxton insisted to the head of the PHS venereal disease division that the agency risked public condemnation by continuing the racist trial (Jones 1993). PHS officials worried about public perception amid the civil rights protests of the time, and convened a blue-ribbon panel to review whether to continue the study. Again, however, the panel focused on maximizing the scientific value of the work, and recommended that the project continue. When PHS officials contacted Buxton in 1970 to report on the panel's findings, he began to discuss his ethical and legal concerns with others. Ultimately, in July 1972, Buxton provided his papers and correspondence to a friend who worked as a reporter with the AP wire service. She, in turn, passed them to Jean Heller in AP's Washington, D.C., bureau, who found the PHS willing to confirm every aspect of Buxton's story. Heller's exposé prompted an avalanche of media attention that raised the specter of Nazi research and government-sponsored racism, forcing an end to the study in 1973.

The Tuskegee Syphilis Study Ad Hoc Advisory Panel, convened the day after the AP story broke, concluded in 1973 that "(I)n retrospect, the Public Health Service Study of Untreated Syphilis in the Male Negro in Macon County, Alabama, was ethically unjustified in 1932" (Tuskegee Syphilis Study 1973). The crux of this charge lay in the absence of evidence that study subjects had consented to participate in research, or that they had any knowledge of the risk that the study presented to their own lives as well as to others whom they may have infected during the course of the trial. Moreover, the panel also found the study to be "scientifically unsound," based on its lack of a written protocol, the variability of the research questions over the course of the study, and the lack of standardized procedures and evaluation over the 40-year period.

In response to the panel report and the public uproar over the PHS' lack of ethical concern for research subjects, Senator Edward Kennedy convened hearings on human experimentation that led to the federal protections mandated by the National Research Act of 1974 and the creation of the National Commission for the Protection of Human Subjects of Biomedical and Behavioral Research. The Commission's cornerstone document, The Belmont Report (The National Commission for the Protection of Human Subjects of Biomedical and Behavioral Research 1978), laid out the principles of respect for persons, beneficence, and justice as the underpinnings of all legitimate medical research. It further stipulated that the processes of informed consent, risk/benefit assessment, and the selection of subjects must be conducted with careful attention to the demands of these principles.

In the three decades since the end of the Tuskegee Syphilis Study, governmental attention to the ethical oversight of research, researchers' own growing awareness of the ethical tensions in their work, and the development of the field of bioethics have fostered steady interest in the rights and protection of research subjects. However, in the 1970s and 1980s, efforts to protect vulnerable populations from the risks of research often led to their exclusion altogether, in favor of research on young White men assumed to provide an adequate picture of the wider human experience of disease and its treatment (Dresser 1992). Although the National Institutes of Health (NIH) subsequently imposed formal requirements on federally funded research to include minorities and women in research on conditions that affect them disproportionately (National Institutes of Health and Alcohol, Drug Abuse, and Mental Health Administration 1990), Tuskegee's profound legacy has been the continued disparity in health status between Whites and Blacks. African-Americans' distrust of medical and public health professionals has affected not only their access to care, but also the extent of research on health problems affecting African-Americans (Gamble 1997).

As noted by Patricia A. King, a health law scholar who served on the original National Commission, both recognizing and ignoring racial differences may have dangerous consequences for the health of minority populations (King 1992). The dilemma lies in how to recognize the correlations between race and disease. While it is important to recognize individual groups' special needs and the effects of past injustices, such recognition must avoid reinforcing negative stereotypes and prevent the indirect harms that may arise from well-intentioned efforts to enhance health. Thus the dilemma of difference remains one of the greatest conceptual and practical challenges for the future of ethical biomedical research.

The Dilemma of Difference in Current Debates on Research Ethics

The AZT Trials and International Standards of Consent

Following The Belmont Report's careful articulation of the principles underlying the ethics of biomedical research—respect for persons, beneficence, and justice—ethical principles have been at the center of much of medical ethics over the past two decades. Part of the appeal of principalism is the belief that it is possible to identify universal ethical principles and related mandates for ethical behavior that apply in any context. One such ethical mandate, stemming from the principle of respect for persons, is the requirement for informed consent found in the Nuremberg Code, the Declaration of Helsinki, and all U.S. regulations governing research. A second is the requirement laid out in the Declaration of Helsinki that therapeutic research proceed only from the point of clinical equipoise, and that all subjects—including controls—receive nothing less than the standard of care (Freedman 1987).

Beginning in the 1980s, experience in international research gradually began to call into question the western interpretation of individual autonomy and social justice that lay behind these requirements (Angell 1988; Barry 1988; Levine 1992). The emergence of HIV/AIDS was a major factor in the renewal of international debate about research ethics. By the mid-1990s antiretroviral treatment was the standard of care in North America and Europe, but new cases of HIV infection were already appearing disproportionately in developing countries where there were no affordable therapeutic options. Treatment and research efforts directed toward Asia and Africa often created new uncertainties about informed consent and the meaning of "standard of care." In 1993, the World Health Organization (WHO) and the Council for International Organizations of Medical Sciences (CIOMS) provided a baseline for international research ethics, asserting that the ethical standards applied to research in developing countries should be "no less exacting" than those that would be used if the study were conducted in the researchers' or sponsors' own country (World Health Organization 1993). But as hundreds of thousands of people unable to afford HIV drugs died, rapid development of a less expensive effective intervention became a top priority.

The already spirited professional debate on international ethical standards exploded in 1997 when two physicians with the Public Citizen's Health Research Group denounced several studies on the perinatal transmission of HIV in developing countries in a report in the *New England Journal of Medicine* (Lurie and Wolfe 1997). Drs. Peter Lurie and Sidney M. Wolfe reported that in 15 of 16 protocols designed to assess interventions to reduce the perinatal transmission of HIV in African countries where AZT was prohibitively expensive, some or all of the subjects were denied the standard of care as part of placebo-controlled trials. Noting that a number of these studies were underwritten by NIH and CDC, Lurie and Wolfe condemned the use of placebo controls as a breach of U.S. regulations and international ethical standards that would lead to the needless infection and deaths of hundreds of infants. They rejected researchers' contention that placebo treatment could be considered the standard of care in developing countries because it was equal to or better than what the subjects would have received had they not been part of the protocol. They also took issue with an implied double standard that created an incentive to do expensive research in countries where potential subjects might be coerced into participation by their limited access to care and their need for treatment.

Where the essay by Lurie and Wolfe was provocative, calling NIH and CDC unethical for their financial support and encouragement of placebo-controlled AZT trials, the accompanying editorial by Dr. Marcia Angell was even more critical. Angell accused the researchers and federal agencies of a "callous disregard" for the welfare of the study subjects (Angell 1997). Angell repeated the charge made by the Public Citizen's Health Research Group that the U.S. funded placebo-control research was exploitation of people of color (Lurie 1997), and drew parallels between the agencies' ethical relativism in the African AZT studies and their disregard for African-American subjects in the Tuskegee Syphilis Study. Her remarks ignited a public controversy that renewed debate about the syphilis trial and sparked a sometimes rancorous exchange with government health officials and NIH-sponsored AIDS researchers about how best to reduce the spread of AIDS in developing countries.

Dr. Harold Varmus, head of NIH, and Dr. David Satcher, head of CDC, published an editorial in response to Angell that insisted that the studies in question had been subjected to rigorous ethical review and were conducted in keeping with widely accepted ethical principles and guidelines (Varmus and Satcher 1997). Ultimately, they argued, the need for definitive scientific answers and a clear view of side effects made placebo-controlled trials the best way to provide useful knowledge to the subjects and others in the population. Angell remained unconvinced, and repeated the comparison between the African research and Tuskegee in a public appeal in the lay press (Angell 1997).

Lurie and Wolfe and other research physicians and ethicists called for a "careful, global dialogue" (Lurie and Wolfe 1997) and "extensive public discussion" (Faden and Kass 1998) on how international medical research should address differences in standards of care and the constraints on informed consent where research offered the only available treatment. In 1997 and 1998, WMA and CIOMS again took up the ethics of international research, debating whether and how to re–revise the Declaration of Helsinki and the International Ethical Guidelines to address developing countries' contemporary medical needs and financial exigencies (Levine 1999). Proponents of revising the provisions on equipoise and placebo controls insisted that international standards had to change to recognize impoverished nations' desperate need for new, affordable medications. Critics feared that change would lead to a more rapid expansion of research in areas where the higher rates of disease, lower standards of care, and power differentials between researchers and subjects would lead to the exploitation of the world's poor by wealthier countries and the pharmaceutical industry (Faden and Kass 1998; Brennan 1999; Lurie and Wolfe 1999).

After extensive debate among members of the WMA and professional and public commentary via a dedicated Internet website, the WMA adopted the sixth revised version of the Declaration of Helsinki on October 2000 at its annual meeting in Edinburgh, Scotland. The new edition modified the stipulation that every patient–subject, including members of control groups, receive "the best proven diagnostic and therapeutic methods," to call for every patient–subject to receive "*proven effective* prophylactic, diagnostic, and therapeutic methods," (emphasis added) (World Medical Association 2000). The new version also provided for the use of a placebo where no proven diagnostic or therapeutic method exists.

In December 1998, as the WMA addressed international research controversies, CIOMS also undertook revision of its International Ethical Guidelines. Although the discussion was less public than the WMA's concensus-building process, professional debate was nonetheless vigorous. Several rounds of commentary by steering committee members and authors of commissioned papers on proposed revisions led to the December 2000 publication of *Biomedical Research Ethics: Updating International Guidelines (A Consultation)*, redrafted versions in June 2001 and January 2002, and a CIOMS conference the following month. At the conference, dispute regarding the legitimacy of placebo controls continued in debate over the text of Guideline 11, "Choice of Control in Clinical Trials." Ultimately, this conflict could not be resolved, and a commentary was added that detailed the opposing ethical positions regarding the comparisons with all but established effective intervention (Council for International Organizations of Medical Sciences 2002).

Notably, in professional guidelines and theoretical discourse, early attention to racial injustices in international trials has all but given way to concern for economic disparities between rich and poor countries. In particular, Angell's charge that placebo-controlled AZT research revisited the abuses of Tuskegee seems to have had a chilling effect on the consideration of race in the exploitation of research subjects. Ethicist Ronald Bayer condemned the reference to Tuskegee as an "exploitation of racism" in an arena where the real moral issue is the "maldistribution of wealth and resources" (Bayer 1998). Ruth Faden and Nancy Kass likewise contended that, in dealing with the challenge of research in resource–poor environments, analogies to Tuskegee "distract from a critical and honest dialogue" (Faden and Kass 1998). Although no one explicitly denies the possibility that racism affects international research, U.S. commentators appear to be more comfortable focusing debate on the effects of poverty. Nonetheless, as the regulation of international research prompts attention to the real risks of economic exploitation, how race and racism affect national and international economies must be part of the equation. The challenge will be to recognize the effects and persistence of racism in national and international economic disparities and, more importantly, to determine how to redress them in current research policy.

The Human Genome Diversity Project and the Genetic Definition of Race

Beyond the boom in international research prompted by HIV/AIDS, biomedical research at the turn of the millennium has also been characterized by rapid developments in genetics. As the most significant "big science" project in decades, the Human Genome Project's map of the human genome not only offers an opportunity to understand the genetic factors in health and illness, it promises to reveal important genetic information about the human condition in general. In 1990 Stanford population geneticist Luigi Luca Cavalli-Szforza proposed a project to complement the Human Genome Project, the creation of a database of genetic information about the world's distinct human populations, intended to improve understanding of the full scope of human variation (Cavalli-Sforza 1990). This endeavor, subsequently called the Human Genome Diversity Project (HGDP), has met with international controversy over the meaning of genetic information, the nature of community identity, and the role of racism in genetics and genetic research.

The HGDP began in 1991 with the goal of collecting DNA samples and cultural information from 500 of the world's 4000–8000 distinct human groups. The official HGDP website at Stanford University's Morrison Institute for Population and Resource Studies describes the project as an international effort that "seeks to understand the diversity and unity of the entire human species (Human Genome Diversity Project)." HGDP's organizers anticipate that their HGDP database will help researchers understand the processes of evolution and the complex nature of many human characteristics, including that of ethnicity. Moreover, they expect their data to highlight what is already known about human interrelatedness, that there is more genetic variation among the members of any one ethnic group than exists between different groups (Human Genome Diversity Project). Cavalli-Szforza and his colleagues have argued that HGDP will ultimately reduce the threat of racism worldwide by documenting the fact the concept of race as a fundamental biological category is flawed (Butler 1995).

HGDP was originally funded with $500,000 in seed money from private foundations and planning grants from the U.S. government. In 1994 it formalized its affiliation with the nonprofit scientific group known as the Human Genome Organization (HUGO), which appointed an international executive committee to oversee the project's work. Regional committees for North America, Europe, Eastern and Southeastern Asia, Australia and the Pacific, India, China, Central and South America, and Africa are responsible for fundraising and overseeing data collection. This structure is intended to enhance the project's sensitivity to regional issues and to address the concerns of the particular peoples of each respective region (Human Genome Diversity Project, Frequently Asked Questions).

Since its inception, HGDP has met with criticism about ethical issues in its proposed research, particularly from advocacy groups representing indigenous populations concerned about exploitation and abuse. In 1994, HGDP sought the backing of the United Nations Educational Scientific and Cultural Organization (UNESCO), but a working group on population genetics established by UNESCO's International Bioethics Committee (IBC) rejected the request for endorsement and funding in 1995 (Butler 1995). The subcommittee's report particularly addressed the fears of indigenous peoples regarding stigmatization and discrimination resulting from inclusion in the database, and possible eugenics related to the interpretation of HGDP's data by others (Subcommittee on Bioethics and Population Genetics of the UNESCO International Bioethics Committee 1995). Moreover, the report was also critical of HGDP's basic approach to the study of indigenous people; it was unclear how the project would benefit the groups sampled or how the researchers would address intellectual property rights to the sampled DNA.* Advocates for indigenous peoples took the criticism to an even more basic level, arguing that the science of genetics vio-

---

* Intellectual property rights to DNA became an issue independent of the HGDP because of the work of researchers with NIH and CDC who sought to patent the donated DNA of three members of indigenous populations from Papua New Guinea, Panama, and the Solomon Islands. The individuals' communities and other groups insisted that the donors' consent for the original research had never included the issue of patient rights since their cultures did not accept the concept of the ownership of nature.

lated the holistic worldview of many cultures in which human origins are a sacred part of ancient mythology.

The IBC was particularly doubtful of the claim that HGDP data would reduce the risk of racism, arguing instead that "racism is an attitude that may seek its justification in science" (Subcommittee on Bioethics and Population Genetics of the UNESCO International Bioethics Committee 1995). Despite HGDP's intent to provide morally neutral information, the committee feared that others might assume that genetic differences provide a basis for labels of "superior" and "inferior," and insisted that it was naive to presume that scientists themselves cannot be racist. Finally, they concluded, "It is very important to realise that scientific information, in and of itself, is never likely to significantly undermine race as a political category or eugenics as a political and social movement" (Subcommittee on Bioethics and Population Genetics of the UNESCO International Bioethics Committee 1995).

HGDP subsequently pursued funding from NIH and the National Science Foundation (NSF), which commissioned a review of the project by the National Academy of Sciences (NAS) in 1996 (Kreeger 1996). A variety of scientists and lay people testified, including several groups of indigenous peoples and representatives of advocacy groups. Indigenous peoples in North, Central, and South America expressed their opposition to HGDP based on a variety of grounds, including the historical experience of western colonialization: "the agenda of the non-indigenous forces has been to appropriate and manipulate the natural order for the purposes of profit, power, and control" (Declaration of Indigenous Peoples of the Western Hemisphere Regarding the Human Genome Diversity Project 1996). Although the NAS panel agreed that human genetic diversity is an important area for multidisciplinary study, it recommended against federal funding until the project's specific research questions, international organizational structure, and related ethical issues could be better defined and resolved (MacIlwain 1997).

To address the concerns of indigenous peoples opposed to HGDP, and to create ethical safeguards for the process of DNA collection, the North American Regional Committee drafted a Model Ethical Protocol for Collecting DNA Samples (North American Regional Committee, Human Genome Diversity Project 1997). The guidelines address making contact with the population to be recruited; informed consent; providing benefits to the participating groups; providing medical services to participating groups; protection of privacy and confidentiality; education and racism; ownership and control of genetic and cultural data; and the creation of partnerships with participating groups in all stages of research. However, although the international executive committee of HGDP has addressed many of the ethical and organizational issues that were identified as barriers to governmental research funding, the project's North American work remains stalled without external support (Smaglik 2000). Related work in other regions has proceeded, with Chinese collaborators already reporting on findings from samples taken from 28 of the 56 ethnic groups officially recognized by the Chinese government (Smaglik 2000; Chu et al. 1998).

The HGDP illustrates the profound ethical tensions inherent in the study of human biological difference as a scientific question. A comprehensive understanding of ethnicity requires both a joint and separate study of genetics and culture. Yet, research into human genetic variability cannot remain value-neutral, as cultural values previously attributed to biological differences will shape interpretation of any findings. If concern for the consequences of the cultural interpretation of difference prevent the research that clarifies genetic distinctions, racist views of difference will be much harder to eliminate and the essential roles of variability will be much harder to recognize. The challenge is to resolve the dilemma of difference through both science and ethics, and to work creatively with the tension while doing so.

Conclusions

The history of modern medical research is a complex tapestry of remarkable technological breakthroughs and life-saving therapeutic advances, dotted with unimaginable abuses and polarizing ethical controversies over the definition of wrongdoing. Painful as they are to revisit, examination of these abuses and the culture of research that permitted them offers many lessons for present-day investigators and ethicists.

The first of these lessons is that science and medicine cannot be value-free. Excellent research demands dedication to the objectivity, skepticism, and critical analysis essential to the scientific method. However, the social, cultural, and political context in which research is conducted inherently shapes the truth upon which the research questions are framed, the identification and definition of key variables, and the ends that research is meant to serve. While it is often easy to spot the effects of prejudice and ideology in the work of previous generations, it is often difficult to recognize these forces as a project is conceived, developed, and carried out. Researchers must be willing to recognize the inherent potential for bias in their ongoing work and acknowledge how such biases may affect the welfare of their human subjects.

A second, related lesson is that, historically, scientific attempts to identify and understand racial differences have been influenced by the pervasive human tendency to view differences among groups as indicative of their relative worth in a natural moral hierarchy. Consideration of the scope of abuse of human subjects reveals that racism may significantly affect the work of researchers who define their own group to be the human "standard" from which others deviate. Thus, research on apparent health-related differences between groups and the meaning of those differences is inherently at risk of incorporating racist perspectives into its questions and methods. While neither specific definitions of racial identity nor the concept of race itself is inherently racist, there remains a risk that subtle forms of racism will affect efforts to study the health of individuals and groups when race is used as a variable. Nonetheless, excluding racial identity from the variables used to understand health and illness may make the significant problems of racial and ethnic minorities invisible to others.

A third lesson is that the potential for racism within science increases the vulnerability of research subjects from some racial and ethnic groups in ways that may not be amenable to regulatory protections. Since the Nuremberg Tribunal established fundamental ethical standards for research with human subjects over 50 years ago, increased regulation, both in society at large and in science and medicine, has significantly reduced the threat of overt racist practices in medical care and research. Nonetheless, as recent debates about U.S. research in developing countries have demonstrated, regulation is almost never specific enough nor broad enough to prevent new and subtle expressions of racism from emerging. Regulation can provide a baseline for ethical action, but mere compliance with formal policies seldom fosters the atmosphere of trust between subjects and researchers that is essential to meeting contemporary ethical ideals.

Moving beyond accusations of wrongdoing and racism to promote collaboration and trust will require good-faith engagement with the ethical significance of race and racism in research and in society at large. Working within the tensions of the dilemma of difference requires researchers and ethicists to openly examine their individual beliefs about race, to listen carefully and with respect to the views, experiences, and needs of the populations that they wish to study, and to engage their colleagues and institutions in a discussion of the ethics that inform their work with all human subjects.

References

Angell M. Ethical imperialism? Ethics in international collaborative clinical research. *N Engl J Med*. 1988;319:1081-2.

Angell M. The ethics of clinical research in the third world. *N Engl J Med*. 1997;337:847-9.

Angell M. Tuskegee revisited. *Wall Street Journal*. Oct. 28, 1997;Sect A(col.3).

Barry M. Ethical considerations of human investigation in developing countries: the AIDS dilemma. *N Engl J Med*. 1988;319:1083-6.

Bayer R. The debate over maternal-fetal HIV transmission prevention trials in Africa, Asia, and the Caribbean: racist exploitation or exploitation of racism? *Am J Public Health*. 1998;88:567-70.

Beecher HK. Ethics and clinical research. *N Engl J Med*. 1966;274:1354-60.

Bernard C. An introduction to experimental medicine. In: Reiser SJ, Dyck AJ, Curran WJ, eds. Ethics in medicine: historical perspectives and contemporary concerns. Cambridge, Mass.: MIT Press; 1978;257.

Bordley J, Harvey AMcG. *Two centuries of American medicine: 1776-1976*. Philadelphia: W.B. Saunders Co.; 1976.

Brennan TA. Proposed revisions to the Declaration of Helsinki—will they weaken the ethical principles underlying human research? *N Engl J Med*. 1999;341:527-31.

Butler D. Genetic diversity proposal fails to impress international ethics panel. *Nature*. 1995;377:373.

Cavalli-Sforza LL. The Chinese Human Genome Diversity Project. *Proc Natl Acad Sci*. 1998; 95:11501-3.

Cavalli-Sforza LL. Opinion: How can one study individual variation for 3 billion nucleotides of the human genome? *Am J Hum Genetics*. 1990;46:649-51.

Chu JY, Huang W, Kuang SQ, Wang JM, Xu JJ, Chu ZT, Yang ZQ, et al. Genetic relationship of populations in China. *Proc Natl Acad Sci*. 1998;95:11763-8.

Council for International Organizations of Medical Sciences. International ethical guidelines for biomedical research involving human subjects. Geneva: IOMS. 2002. Available at: http://www.cioms.ch.

Declaration of indigenous peoples of the western hemisphere regarding the Human Genome Diversity Project, 1996 (Feb 8). Available at: http://www.whitestareagle.com/natlit/ genome.htm.

Dower JW. *Embracing defeat: Japan in the wake of World War II*. New York: W.W. Norton & Co.; 1999.

Dresser R. Wanted: single white male for medical research. *Hastings Ctr Rep*. 1992:22 (Jan-Feb): 24-29.

Endicott S, Hagerman E. *The United States and biological warfare: secrets from the early cold war and Korea*. Bloomington, Ind.: University of Indiana Press; 1998.

Faden R, Kass N. HIV research, ethics, and the developing world. *Am J Public Health*. 1998;88:548-50.

Freedman B. Equipoise and the ethics of clinical research. *N Engl J Med*. 1987;317:141-5.

Gamble VN. Under the shadow of Tuskegee: African Americans and health care. *Am J Public Health*. 1997;87:1773-7.

Girdwood RH. Medicine and the media: Experimentation on prisoners by the Japanese during World War II. *Brit Med J*. 1985; 291(6494):530-1.

Gold H. *Unit 731 testimony: Japan's wartime human experimentation program*. Singapore: Yenbooks; 1996.

Goldhagen DJ. *Hitler's willing executioners: ordinary Germans and the Holocaust*. New York: Vintage Books; 1997.

Harris S. *Factories of death: Japanese biological warfare, 1932-1945, and the American cover-up*. London: Routledge; 1994.

Hornblum AM. *Acres of skin: human experiments at Holmsburg Prison. A true story of abuse and exploitation in the name of medical science*. New York: Routledge; 1998.

Howard-Jones N. Human experimentation in historical and ethical perspective. *Soc Sci Med*. 1982;16:1429-48.

Human Genome Diversity Project. Available at: http://www.stanford.edu/group/morrisnt/HGDP.html.

Human Genome Diversity Project. Frequently asked questions. Available at: http://www.stanford.edu/group/morrisnt/hgdp/faq.html.

Ivy AC. Nazi war crimes of a medical nature. *Fed Bull*. 1947;33:133-46. (In: Reiser SJ, Dyck AJ, Curran WJ, eds. *Ethics in medicine: historical perspectives and contemporary concerns*. Cambridge, Mass.: MIT Press; 1978:267-72.)

Jones J. *Bad blood: the Tuskegee syphilis experiment*. New York: The Free Press; 1993.

Jones J. Race and medicine. In: Reich WT, ed. *Encyclopedia of bioethics*. Vol. 4. New York: The Free Press; 1978:1405-10.

King PA. The dangers of difference. *Hastings Ctr Rep*. 1992;22(Nov-Dec):35-8.

Kreeger KY. Proposed Human Genome Diversity Project still plagued by controversy and questions. *Scientist*. 1996;10(20):1,8. Available at: http://www.the-scientist.lib.upenn.edu/yr1996/oct.kreeger_p1_961014.html.

Lederer S. Hideyo Noguchi's luetin experiment and the antivivisectionists. *Isis*. 1985;76:31-48.

Levine RJ. Informed consent: some challenges to the universal validity of the western model. *Law Med Health Care*. 1992;19:207-13.

Levine RJ. The need to revise the Declaration of Helsinki. *N Engl J Med*. 1999;341:531-4.

Lifton RJ. *The Nazi doctors: medical killing and the psychology of genocide*. New York: Basic Books; 1986.

Lurie P. Open letter to DHHS Secretary Donna Shalala. Apr. 22, 1997. Available at: http://www.citizen.org/hrg/publications/1493.htm.

Lurie P, Wolfe SM. Scientists seek to justify and continue unethical research by gutting international ethical guidelines. Public Citizen press release, Aug. 11, 1999. Available at: http://www.citizen.org/hrg/publications/1493.htm

Lurie P, Wolfe SM. Unethical trials of interventions to reduce perinatal transmission of the human immunodeficiency virus in developing countries. *N Engl J Med*. 1997;337:853-6.

MacIlwain C. Diversity project does not merit federal funding. *Nature*. 1997;398:774.

Moe K. Should the Nazi research data be cited? *Hastings Ctr Rep*. 1984;14(Dec):5-7.

The National Commission for the Protection of Human Subjects of Biomedical and Behavioral Research. The Belmont report: Ethical principles for the protection of human subjects of research. Washington, D.C.: U.S. Government Printing Office; 1978.

National Institutes of Health and Alcohol, Drug Abuse, and Mental Health Administration. Special instruction to applicants using form PHS 398 regarding implementation of the NIH/ADAMHA Policy concerning Inclusion of Women and Minorities in Clinical Research Study Populations. Washington, D.C.: NIH; December 1990.

North American Regional Committee, Human Genome Diversity Project. Proposed model ethical protocol for collecting DNA samples. *Houston Law Rev*. 1997;33:1431-73. Available at: http://www.stanford.edu/group/morrisnt/hgdp/protocol.html.

Nuland SB. *Doctors: the biography of medicine*. New York: Vintage Books; 1988.

The Nuremberg Code. In: Trials of war criminals before the Nuremberg Military Tribunals under Control Council Law No. 10. Vol. 2. Washington, D.C.: U.S. Government Printing Office; 1949:181-2. In: Reiser SJ, Dyck AJ, Curran WJ, eds. *Ethics in medicine: historical perspectives and contemporary concerns*. Cambridge, Mass.: MIT Press; 1978:272-3.

Powell JW. Japan's biological weapons, 1930-1945: a hidden chapter in history. *Bull Atomic Sci.* 1981;37(8):43-53.

Powell JW. Japan's germ warfare: the U.S. Cover-up of a War Crime. *Bull Concerned Asian Scholars.* 1980;12(2):2-17.

Proctor RN. *The Nazi war on cancer*. Princeton, N.J.: Princeton University Press; 1999.

Rothman DJ. *Strangers at the bedside: a history of how law and bioethics transformed medical decision making*. New York: Basic Books; 1991.

Schwitalla AM. The real meaning of research and why it should be encouraged. *Mod Hosp.* 1929; 33(4):77-80. In Reiser SJ, Dyck AJ, Curran WJ, eds. *Ethics in medicine: historical perspectives and contemporary concerns*. Cambridge, Mass.: MIT Press; 1978: 264-6.

Smaglik P. Genetic diversity project fights for its life [news]. *Nature.* 2000, 404:912.

Subcommittee on Bioethics and Population Genetics of the UNESCO International Bioethics Committee. Bioethics and human population genetics research. Final report. Paris: UNESCO; 1995 (Nov 15). Available from: URL:http://www.biol.tsukuba.ac.jp~macer/PG.htm.

Thompson A. Former slave laborers for Nazis hold protest. *Houston Chronicle.* March 26, 1999;Sect A:30(col 1).

Tuskegee Syphilis Study Ad Hoc Advisory Panel. Final report. Washington, D.C.: U.S. Public Health Service; 1973.

U.S. Public Health Service. Division of Research Grants. Clinical investigations involving human subjects. Memo PPO #129, Feb. 8, 1966 and supplement, Apr. 7, 1966. Washington, D.C.: U.S. Public Health Service.

Varmus H, Satcher D. Ethical complexities of conducting research in developing countries. *N Engl J Med.* 1997;337:1003-5.

Weiss J. *Ideology of death: why the Holocaust happened in Germany*. Chicago, Ill.: Ivan R. Dee; 1996.

Withington CF. The possible conflict between the interests of medical science and those of the individual patient, and the latter's indefeasible rights. In: *The relation of hospitals to medical education*. Boston: Cupples, Uphman and Co.; 1886:14-17. In: Reiser SJ, Dyck AJ, Curran WJ, eds. *Ethics in medicine: historical perspectives and contemporary concerns*. Cambridge, Mass.: MIT Press; 1978:260-1.

World Health Organization. International ethical guidelines for biomedical research involving human subjects. Geneva: Council for International Organizations of Medical Science; 1993.

World Medical Association. Declaration of Helsinki: recommendations guiding medical doctors in biomedical research involving human subjects. Geneva: WMA; 2000; Available at: http://www.wma.net.

Chapter 4

CLINICAL TRIALS

Neil R. Powe, MD, MPH, MBA,
and Tiffany L. Gary, PhD

Description of Clinical Trials

From a scientific perspective, clinical trials are the most rigorous type of studies. In the past few decades clinical trials have emerged as the "gold standard" in the evaluation of medical treatments and interventions (Friedman, Furberg, and Demets 1998). The purpose of this chapter is to define clinical trials, briefly review their methods of conduct and design, discuss standard approaches to recruitment and retention, and present historical evidence of the misuse of clinical trials with ethnic minorities.

Definition

A clinical trial is a study design used in epidemiology and clinical research studies to assess how the health outcomes associated with one type of intervention (or exposure) administered to one group of persons compares to another intervention given to a comparable group of persons. The health outcomes, survival, morbidity, symptoms, quality of life, or resource utilization can be measured over a short time or many years. The interventions can be a screening practice, a preventive approach, a diagnostic strategy, or a treatment regimen. When no intervention is administered or routine circumstances are used in the group for comparison, we refer to the intervention as a placebo. Because investigators in clinical trials purposely assign interventions to subjects, clinical trials are often referred to as experimental rather than observational studies.

Observational studies differ from experimental studies in that investigators observe persons who have already received different interventions administered in the course of routine practice rather than those deliberately assigned by an investigator. There are different types of observational studies including cohort studies, case-control studies, and cross-sectional studies. In a cohort study, groups of individuals with different exposures are followed over time for an outcome of interest. In a case-control study, subjects are selected (or assembled) for study based on their achievement of a particular outcome; exposure to a risk factor or intervention is then ascertained among those with the outcome and those without the outcome. In cross-sectional studies, the relation is assessed between exposures and outcomes that are measured simultaneously. Although all of these observational studies are valuable in scientific inquiry, they have limitations, the most important of which is potential bias in selection of the groups that receive intervention, a circumstance that is overcome in clinical trials by random allocation of the intervention to subjects. Also, temporal relationships between the exposures and outcomes in case-control and cross-sectional studies are nearly impossible to disentangle.

Allocation of the intervention to the groups in a clinical trial can be performed in different ways: at the individual level or in groups defined by time or setting (e.g., treated on a given day of the week, managed on one inpatient unit or another). The latter way, in groups, is often defined as quasi-experimental. When persons are assigned to different interventions by chance, the clinical trial is often referred to as a randomized clinical trial; random number generators often are used to decide which persons will be exposed to the intervention and which persons will not.

Clinical trials, particularly for testing of new drugs, have been classified into four phases. In Phase I trials, investigators test an intervention in a small number of subjects (typically less than 100) for the first time to evaluate its safety, determine the ranges of doses, and identify important side effects. In Phase II trials, the intervention is given to a larger number of subjects (typically in the range of 100–300) to see if it is efficacious. Safety also continues to be investigated. In Phase III studies, the intervention is given to even larger numbers of subjects (typically in the range 1,000–3,000) to substantiate efficacy and safety compared to commonly used interventions. Less common side effects are also investigated in the larger group of subjects. Investigators also collect additional information that will allow the intervention to be applied in a safe fashion. In Phase IV trials, the interventions are studied after the market launch of the intervention. Such Phase IV studies typically assess effectiveness in thousands of patients and identify and quantify the less common and prolonged-use side effects in routine practice.

Clinical trials can be performed in a single institution or can be conducted in many institutions (i.e., multicenter clinical trials). Single-institution trials are inherently easier to conduct as they involve policies and investigators at a single institution. Multicenter clinical trials are more complex because standardized procedures must be adapted to many institutions that may vary in research infrastructure, expertise, operations, and culture. However, multicenter trials are usually more generalizable in that they represent a broader segment of the participants or health care providers to whom the results might apply and have the advantage of more rapid recruitment of a large number of participants.

Steps in the Performance of a Clinical Trial

Clinical trials require a great deal of effort in planning, implementation, surveillance, and analysis. Procedures must be established for recruitment of subjects, to see if recruited subjects meet entry criteria, and to determine how eligible subjects will be enrolled. Decisions must also be made on how interventions will be allocated to enrolled patients as well as the procedures to be established on how measurements will be made, how subjects will be followed for outcomes, and, finally, how the data will be analyzed. In regard to minority participation in clinical trials, procedures on recruitment and follow-up are very important to ensure full participation of individuals in clinical trials. The steps or stages of a clinical trial include the design, protocol development, recruitment, intervention implementation, follow-up, patient closeout, and termination (Meinert 1986). These will be briefly described.

Design

Early design of a clinical trial involves specification of many important issues. First, the goals and aims must be enumerated and translated into testable hypotheses that guide the primary and secondary measures for the study. In addition, design includes specification of the number and type of interventions and control groups; issues such as the dose, frequency, and duration of the intervention; and how the interventions will be allocated. Participant stratification during allocation of the intervention is often used to achieve balance of characteristics between intervention groups. Designs should also indicate whether participants (and/or care providers) will be blinded from the knowledge of who will or will not receive the intervention. The primary outcome (e.g., survival) and secondary outcomes (e.g., change in a laboratory measure, hospitalization) need to be defined in light of clinical salience, feasibility, and sample size considerations. The frequency (e.g., every 3 months) and duration (e.g., 2 years) of observations along with how they will be made (e.g., laboratory, medical record review, questionnaire) should be specified. The number of participants (sample size) and study centers needed in order to achieve adequate statistical power is another important part of early design. Participant selection criteria, including eligibility and exclusion criteria, need to be specified and the rules for terminating participants from the trial must be defined. Organizational structure (especially for large multicenter clinical trials) must be designed and should include the use of safety and monitoring committees, which ensure that subjects suffer no harm through their participation in a clinical trial. Recruitment, intervention and data collection procedures, data processing, and data analysis plans also need to be specified.

Protocol Development

Development of the protocol involves creation of a study procedure manual; this is a detailed document that includes specifics on how to identify participants, obtain consent, administer interventions, and collect data within the designated follow-up times. Data-collection forms that document essential information on the application of the intervention, outcomes, and data needed for tracking are designed in protocol development. The details of how study staff will be organized, trained, and communicated with, and how quality of the procedures and data will be guaranteed, are also documented. Documenting how participant confidentiality will be maintained is another important aspect of protocol development.

Recruitment

The goal of recruitment in a clinical trial is to obtain a sufficient number of subjects to have statistical confidence in the results and the confidence in subsequent infer‑ences made based on those results. The requisite numbers of persons needed are deter‑mined through quantitative analyses of the power of the study. Recruitment strate‑gies depend on a variety of considerations, including whether persons being recruited can accurately identify themselves as meeting the eligibility criteria for the study, whether the investigators have access to such individuals, and the resources avail‑able to the study team. Direct recruitment of individuals by investigators can be done through clinic contacts, screenings at public venues, telephone solicitation, direct mailing, and now the Internet. With appropriate authorization, indirect patient recruitment can be done through physicians or other health professionals who are asked to refer appropriate persons to the study; review of medical records from health care providers; analysis of administrative records from health care organizations or insurers; review of clinical databases (such as laboratory test databases); or a combi‑nation of these approaches. Barriers to participation of minorities in clinical trials can occur with a variety of recruitment approaches.

Interventions, Follow-Up, and Retention

This step includes application of the intervention, monitoring to ensure appropri‑ate application with regard to safety, follow‑up of participants, and efforts to retain participants for the full course of the trial. Clinical trials, particularly those lasting for a long period of time, pose a significant challenge to maintaining full participa‑tion of subjects over the life of the study, and attrition of subjects can be trouble‑some for investigators. It may be necessary for the objectives of a clinical trial for researchers to estimate the true incidence of an outcome; losses to follow‑up make this more difficult. In addition, if more individuals in one of the intervention groups are lost to follow‑up than their counterparts in another group, a bias may result due to differential attrition. Approaches to maximizing retention of subjects are an inte‑gral part of the design of the study. For example, subjects may be excluded at the out‑set if they are unlikely to maintain follow‑up and strategies may be employed to ensure vigilant tracking of subjects once they are enrolled. There are a variety of rea‑sons why minorities participating in clinical trials may not have full retention.

Patient Closeout, Termination, Data Analysis, and Reporting

This last step involves procedures for terminating the trial. Final data need to be col‑lected, and study participants need to be informed of which intervention they received in a blinded trial and removed from the intervention (or instructed how they might continue under the intervention either themselves or under the care of a health pro‑fessional). Institutional review boards need to be informed that the trial has ended. Data are analyzed and results of the study are written for publication.

In this chapter, we will address several issues that bear on ensuring that ethnic minorities are made aware of clinical trials, are effectively and ethically enrolled in such studies, and are retained over the life of the study to maximize the information that can be gained from such research. First, we will review historical evidence that may affect attitudes and behaviors of minorities participating in clinical trials. (Chapter 3 by Heitman and Wells includes a detailed examination of historical medical atrocities that have occurred among ethnic minority populations.) Next, we will review national data on participation in clinical trials, and, finally, we will examine the role of participants, investigators, institutions, and funders (see Figure 1) in the full participation of minorities in clinical trials.

Historical Evidence of Deception and Mistrust: Concerns about "Human Experimentation"

African-Americans

African-Americans have a long history of mistrust of the medical community. Although many events throughout slavery triggered mistrust and discrimination, which has persisted since before the civil rights era, the most infamous negative experience involving deception and exploitation was the Tuskegee Syphilis Study.

The Tuskegee Syphilis Study was started during the great Depression in 1932 by the U.S. Public Health Service (Jones 1993). Briefly, it was an observational study that recruited 400 Black men with evidence of syphilis and 200 Black men without the disease to serve as the control group. The primary aim of the study was to evaluate the natural progression of syphilis in African-American men, which was thought to be considerably different than in Caucasian men. Grassroots recruitment methods were used, including collaborating with the Tuskegee Institute, using a Black nurse who was a respected member of the community to facilitate recruitment efforts,

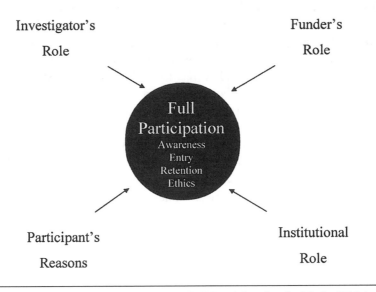

Figure 1. Framework to Achieve Full Participation in Clinical Trials

using churches and schools as sites for data collection, collaborating with plantation owners who employed potential participants, and offering attractive incentives to participants such as transportation, free meals, and burial insurance (Jones 1993).

The true objectives of the study were not communicated to study participants. In fact, the men were not even told that they had syphilis, but instead were told that they had "bad blood," a generic term used at the time for many diseases. Treatment for syphilis was withheld from the affected men even after the implementation of penicillin as the standard of care in 1943. It is particularly disturbing that tremendous efforts were taken throughout the study to ensure that patients would not receive treatment; for example, those men who received penicillin when they enlisted in the military were excluded from the study. Periodically, committees would meet to discuss the ethical nature of the study, but always decided to keep it running. The study was terminated after 40 years, only because it was exposed to the media in 1972 (Thomas and Quinn 1991).

Many historical accounts and commentaries have been published concerning the study, which has continued to fuel the controversy over this research study (Jones 1993; Thomas and Quinn 1991; Gamble 1997; Gamble 1993; Thomas and Curran 1999; Brawley 1998; Talone 1998; Cox 1998; Fairchild and Bayer 1999; Corbie-Smith 1999a). A television movie, "Miss Evers' Boys" has even been created to depict the study, and has been billed as "fiction based on a factual event" (Brawley 1998). Furthermore, recognizing the heinous actions of the study, on May 16, 1997, President Bill Clinton publicly apologized for the Tuskegee Syphilis Study at a White House ceremony (Gamble 1997).

Events from the study are constantly being recounted, not only by potential study participants, but by researchers as well. When the ethical soundness of a particular study is being questioned, the Tuskegee Study often serves as a basis for comparison. Examples include the politically-charged efforts of needle exchange programs in inner cities, blinded seroprevalence studies for HIV infection, and HIV prevention studies in developing countries, which have been compared to Tuskegee and publicly scrutinized (Fairchild and Bayer 1999; Corbie-Smith 1999b; Bowman 1999; Lurie and Wolfe 1999; Caplan and Annas 1999; Angell 2000). Many researchers feel that the legacy of Tuskegee is being abused, therefore minimizing the gravity of current research. Although this study will be forever referenced in history as an event that damaged the relationship between African-Americans and the medical community at large (medical care and research), it should be noted that the Tuskegee Study was not the sole basis for African-Americans' mistrust of medical research.

Gamble has published several articles that allude to other events in history that have contributed substantially to African-Americans' negative perception of health care (Gamble 1997; Gamble 1993). In her articles "Under the Shadow of Tuskegee: African-Americans and Health Care," and "A Legacy of Distrust: African-Americans and Medical Research," she examines several incidents of experimentation on slaves and free Blacks after the Civil War. Examples include medical researchers who forced a slave to sit on a stool on a platform that had been heated to a high temperature five or six times to test remedies for heatstroke (Gamble 1993); the so-called "father of modern gynecology" who subjected three slave women to 30 painful operations in order to develop a technique to repair vesico-vaginal fistulas (Gamble 1993); and folktales of "night doctors," medical students or professional thieves who stole living humans and cadavers from graves and sold them to physicians for medical research (Gamble 1997).

Racial discrimination and stereotypes persisted in public health and medicine through the civil rights era to the present (Charatz-Litt 1992; Reynolds 1997a; Reynolds 1997b; McBride 1993; Menefee 1996; Smith 1998; Rice and Jones 1985). In the 1960s, incidents of discrimination against African-Americans in hospital policies and practices were documented and challenged by civil rights advocates, which led to action by the federal government (Civil Rights Act of 1964, Title VI) (Reynolds 1997a; Reynolds 1997b). In addition, research has perpetuated the notion that there are inherent differences in disease between African-Americans and Whites, although many studies have shown that much of the racial disparity in disease can be explained by socioeconomic status (SES) and other nonracial modifiable factors. Furthermore, in the 1990s, a growing research area has been evaluating access to treatment and differential treatment patterns between racial groups (Schulman et al. 1999; Ayanian et al. 1999; Ayanian et al. 1993; Cooper-Patrick et al. 1999; Ford et al. 1989; Franks et al. 1993; Furth et al. 2000; Giles et al. 1995; Goldberg et al. 1992; Hannan et al. 1991; Johnson et al. 1993; LaVeist, Keith, and Gutierrez 1995; Lozano, Connell, and Koepsell 1995; McBean, Warren, and Babish 1994; Mirvis et al. 1994; Wenneker and Epstein 1989; Whittle et al. 1993). Unfortunately, many of these studies have shown unfavorable outcomes for ethnic minorities. Response to the persistent legacy of discrimination in research and health care is evident in the low study participation rates among African-Americans. Further discussion in this chapter will address barriers to participation and potential solutions to increase participation.

Other Ethnic Minority Populations

Although the historical evidence for distrust of the medical community is less available in other ethnic minority populations, racial discrimination is still an issue. Numerous barriers can be identified to explain the low participation rates of Native American and Hispanic populations in research. For example, cultural practices are often not incorporated into approaches to outreach and medical practice in specific populations. Navajo Indians from northeast Arizona may not share similar attitudes toward health and illness as western physicians (Carey et al. 1991; Carrese and Rhodes 2000). Ho'zho', one of the most important concepts in the Navajo culture, combines the concepts of beauty, goodness, order, harmony, and everything that is positive or ideal (Carrese and Rhodes 1995). The full phrases of the concept are ho'zhooji' nitsihakees and ho'zhooji'saad, which literally translate to "think in the Beauty Way" and "talk in the Beauty Way." It is believed that thought and language have the power to shape reality and control events. This may directly contradict western practices in medicine and research including informed consent, in which patients are notified of their risks. While researchers believe that they are carrying out an ethical obligation to inform patients of potential harms, shaping the discussion in a negative manner may only widen the communication gap between some participants and the medical community.

It is also well known that Hispanics have difficulty utilizing health care services due to many factors, one of the most pronounced being the Spanish–English language barrier (Suarez et al. 1994; Corkery et al. 1996). It has been shown, in the diabetes literature, that the use of bicultural, bilingual Hispanic-American community health workers operating in clinic settings improved rates of completion of a diabetes education program (Corkery et al. 1996). These community health workers attended clinic sessions with patients and served as Spanish-interpreters, reinforced self-care instructions, and reminded patients of upcoming appointments. Researchers should take lessons from these successful programs. Identifying these patterns and implementing culturally sensitive interventions may be the key to increasing participation in health research.

Participation Rates in Various Clinical Trials

Information from Previous Studies

Data regarding minority participation rates in clinical trials are limited. Svensson published a review article that summarized the representation of American Blacks in clinical trials of new drugs (Svensson 1989). The study reviewed all published articles in *Clinical Pharmacology and Therapeutics* in 1984–1986 and found that only 10 of 50 studies provided racial data. After acquiring racial data from authors, 35 studies were included in the review. The proportion of African-American subjects in 23 of the studies was lower than the proportion of African-Americans in the city where the study was conducted. In addition, in 20 of the studies, the proportion of African-Americans was lower than the proportion of African-Americans in the United States. Furthermore, the underrepresentation of Blacks and other minorities limited the ability to conduct sub-analyses to determine the drug response in those populations.

National Institutes of Health Policy on the Inclusion of Women and Minorities as Subjects in Clinical Research

In response to the inadequate participation of minorities in research studies, the National Institutes of Health (NIH) implemented a policy on the inclusion of women and minorities as subjects in clinical research (NIH Outreach Notebook Committee 1994). Chapter III-1 of the policy statement provides an in-depth discourse on the development of the NIH Revitalization Act. The policy, implemented in 1994, was created to ensure that women and minorities and their subpopulations are included in all human research. The policy encourages inclusion with adequate numbers to conduct subgroup analyses and requires official documentation of inclusion to facilitate the monitoring of demographic data of all NIH-funded research. Implementation of the policy has been successful, as indicated by the NIH report that more than 93% of applications involving human subjects complied with the requirement to report women and minority inclusion (Roth et al. 1999). Results from the 1997 report on minority inclusion in Phase III clinical trials are located in Figure 2; both American Indian/Alaska Natives and Asian/Pacific Islander populations represented less than 4% of the subjects researched. Hispanic populations represented 4.1% of subjects; and African-Americans represented the largest percentage of the ethnic minority populations that were studied, with a participation rate of 10.6%. Otherwise, Whites made up 58.1% of subjects studied, and those of other or unknown race made up 24.6%. Based on these results, NIH concluded that substantial numbers of minorities have been enrolled and, therefore, inclusion has been accomplished. Arguably, however, the appropriate level of inclusion might depend on the prevalence of the condition/disease studied in the overall population.

The guidelines were updated in August 2000 to address issues beyond the scope of participant enrollment. The updated guidelines emphasize better planning, conducting, and reporting of subgroup analyses. In particular, they state that if prior evidence suggests outcome differences by subgroups, the research plan should include specific details on how the data will be analyzed according to these subgroups. In addition, NIH strongly encourages that investigators include subgroup analyses emanating from the study in publication submissions, suggesting that these efforts may have an impact on the future inclusion of minorities in research. By explicitly focusing attention on the planning of research studies in government-funded research, minority participation may increase. Although government enhancement may be necessary, it may not be sufficient to achieve full participation by minorities in clinical trials unless participant, investigator, and institutional barriers are addressed.

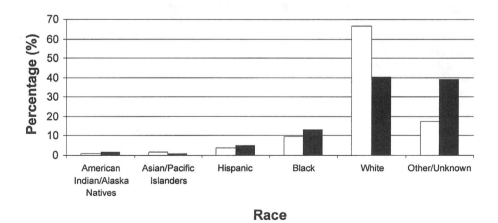

Figure 2. Enrollment in NIH-Funded Extramural Phase III Protocols Funded in Fiscal Year 1997
□ female participation, ■ male participation.
Source: Implementation of the NIH Guidelines on the Inclusion of Women and Minorities as Subjects in Clinical Research: Comprehensive Report (Fiscal Year 1997 Tracking Data).

Barriers to Full Participation

Participants' Roles

Based on a review of the current literature, we have identified potential reasons why minority individuals may not be participating in clinical trials (Roberson 1994; Harris et al. 1996; Shavers-Hornaday et al. 1997; Gorelick et al. 1998; Ballard et al. 1993; Allen 1994; Blumenthal et al. 1995; Corbie-Smith et al. 1999; el Sadr and Capps 1992; Million-Underwood, Sanders, and Davis 1993; Moody et al. 1995; Mouton et al. 1997; Robinson, Ashley, and Haynes 1996; Stoy et al. 1995; Swanson and Ward 1995; Wermeling and Selwitz 1993; Holder et al. 1998). Table 1 summarizes these reasons by outlining each step toward full participation of subjects in clinical trials: awareness, entering, and participation.

Because of the lack of medical resources in minority communities, there may be limited opportunity to learn about clinical trials. Even institutions that are housed within minority communities may not make medical resources fully available or accessible for the surrounding area; however, there have recently been efforts to increase partnerships between clinics and communities as well as implement community outreach and mobilization efforts (Levine, Becker, and Bone 1992; Hatch et al. 1993; Dressler 1993).

During the actual recruitment period, ineffective communication of study objectives by research staff may compromise participation if participants are not clear about the study's intentions. The strong legacy of mistrust among minority communities, previously mentioned, makes explaining every aspect of the study important.

Table 1. Participants' Barriers to Full Participation in Clinical Trials

Barrier	Steps in the Performance of a Clinical Trial		
	Awareness	Recruitment	Retention
Limited opportunity to learn about RCTs	x		
Recruitment schemes	x		
Lack of medical resources in minority communities	x		
Ineffective study staff communication	x	x	x
Language barriers	x	x	x
Mistrust		x	
Negative experience with hospital or injury due to treatment		x	
Family and friends' influence		x	x
Concerns about changing medication		x	
Fatalistic attitudes about chances of recovery from a disease		x	x
Beliefs/moral values		x	x
Religion		x	x
Alternative medicine		x	x
Caring for children or other ill relatives		x	x
Working multiple jobs		x	x
Transportation problems		x	x
Lack of feedback		x	x

Efforts should also be taken to assess cultural factors, such as language barriers, that may impede awareness.

There are also several other barriers that prevent individuals from entering clinical trials. Many minorities have had negative experiences with hospitals, incurred some type of injury due to a particular treatment, or been made aware that their friends or family members have had negative experiences with medicine and research. The importance of oral history as a powerful cultural factor in many communities of color should also be factored in the equation. This is particularly evident in African-American culture where the legacy of the songs and customs of Africa were passed on during slavery through storytelling (Bennet 1991) and, as a result, the longevity of "negative" memories may hinder the recruitment process. Other concerns by a potential participant may be related to living with a particular disease and the subsequent fear of changing medications, especially if the participant is comfortable with his/her treatment plan. Fatalistic attitudes about recovery may also hinder participation in the study if the subject doesn't believe the study will provide him/her with any health benefit. Beliefs and moral values play a large role in the individual's decision to participate in a clinical trial; religious beliefs may discourage certain medications or medical procedures, and beliefs in alternative medicine versus western medicine may also affect potential participants.

Finally, there are various factors that inhibit retention throughout the study: other priorities may take precedence over study obligations; participants may be caring for children or ill relatives, or they may have difficulty attending study visits due to working multiple jobs or problems with transportation. Furthermore, lack of feedback about their progress in the study or the study results may upset participants enough to withdraw from the program.

Investigators' Roles

Investigators can be overly enthusiastic or unnecessarily pessimistic regarding their ability to attain diverse participation in clinical trials. Both new and experienced investigators may be equally enthusiastic about the area they have chosen to study and may believe that all potential participants will see the logic of addressing this important health problem and will come running to enter the study. However, this is seldom the case. Investigators must be prepared to devote considerable effort to make potential participants aware of the importance and goals of the study, and to realize how their participation can help generate new knowledge that will aid future generations. On the other hand, some investigators may refrain from recruitment of minority participants because they believe the effort is not worth it. This type of pessimistic attitude or lack of self-efficacy must be avoided. Not trying or expending too little effort could lead to lost opportunities to gain valuable information about the impact of interventions on members of minority groups.

Balanced with the zeal to recruit subjects from minority groups must be adherence to ethics in the conduct of human research, including the obtainment of informed consent. Potential subjects must not be coerced into participating or misled about the objectives of the study and their role.

Many investigators have limited knowledge about methods to increase potential participants' awareness of the study. In part this is due to limited local training courses in the mechanics of recruitment for research studies. If such courses do not exist, investigators should seek the advice of experienced investigators who have a track record in recruitment of ethnic minorities in research. In multicenter studies, investigators may have the opportunity to work with national experts who have experience with recruitment and retention of subjects. Many of the experiences learned through years of working with special populations can be imparted to both young investigators and experienced investigators who have not worked with ethnic minorities. Experienced investigators often are knowledgeable about the participant barriers described above, are aware of techniques to overcome them, and may know particular community groups from which to seek support and involvement.

One often overlooked local resource may be individuals who have experience in community outreach or marketing in a specific community. Many medical care institutions have established marketing departments whose role is to analyze the environments in which those institutions reside. Marketing departments may know what avenues can be used to reach certain segments of the community and may have demographic data to guide investigators to appropriate communities. Some of these departments often conduct needs assessments, focus groups, or other types of outreach activities to better understand the attitudes and opinions of the populations they serve with regard to care-seeking behaviors. If such expertise resides in a local institution, investigators should avail themselves of it. Investigators can often use some of these same groups to better understand what factors may affect decisions of potential research subjects to participate in a clinical trial.

There may be a tendency of investigators to delegate recruitment efforts to staff without the requisite skills, the appropriate guidance, or a commitment to recruit ethnic minorities. Investigators who are committed to diverse enrollment must make minority recruitment a priority and instill these values in their staff. They must stress the importance of using different strategies to give potential participants the full

Table 2. Investigator Barriers to Full Participation in Clinical Trials

Barrier	Steps in the Performance of a Clinical Trial		
	Awareness	Recruitment	Retention
Limited knowledge about methods to increase awareness	x		
Lack of community liaison efforts	x		x
Ineffective guidance to study staff	x		
Recruitment based on convenience	x		
Study run-in periods and selection processes	x		
Stereotypes/attitudes of investigators	x		
Ineffective informed consent process		x	
Ineffective study staff communication		x	x
Limited knowledge of appropriate retention methods			x
Lack of appropriate participant incentives			x
Lack of feedback		x	

opportunity to understand the study's goals and to make informed decisions about participation.

One explicit way in which minority recruitment goals might be addressed is through study designs that require quotas of enrolled patients based on minority status and stratified or blocked randomization by ethnic group.

Once subjects are enrolled, investigators must work to make sure that they continue to participate. This can be addressed in several ways. Participants often desire feedback about what their participation has achieved. Investigators can provide newsletters or conduct open forums for participants to describe the intermediate results of the study, including publications emanating from their participation as well as plans for the next year. For longitudinal studies, a birthday or holiday card sent once a year can keep participants connected. It may also be necessary to provide participant incentives such as reimbursing travel costs, costs associated with time off from work, or caregiving expenses for dependent children or elders. Once subjects are recruited and enrolled, participant incentives can be crucial in maintaining ongoing enthusiasm and participation in the study.

Institutions' Roles

Health care, research, and educational institutions that are engaged in clinical research have a role and responsibility in the participation of minorities in clinical research. On a general level, these institutions have a responsibility to see that research performed on human subjects by their employees or within their walls undergoes institutional review. An institutional review board must be established and must follow basic Department of Health and Human Services policy for protection of human research subjects. These include the assurance of minimization of risk to human subjects; that risks to subjects are reasonable in relation to anticipated benefits; that selection of subjects is equitable; that informed consent is obtained and documented; that there is ongoing monitoring of the risks to participants; that appropriate provisions are in place to preserve confidentiality; and that coercion does not occur, particularly for vulnerable groups.

Institutions must now take an active role in the education of investigators in the ethical conduct of research including clinical trials. The U.S. Public Health Service as of October 2000 requires research institutions to provide training in the responsible conduct of research to all staff engaged in research or research training with

Table 3. Institutional and Funder Barriers to Full Participation in Each Step of the Clinical Trial

Barrier	Steps in the Performance of a Clinical Trial		
	Awareness	Recruitment	Retention
Lack of investigator incentives	x		
Lack of participant incentives	x		x
Limited control over actions of particular institutions	x		x
Institutional stereotypes/attitudes	x		

Public Health Service funds. Each institution applying for or receiving a grant, contract, or cooperative agreement under the Public Health Service Act for either research or research training must certify that the institution has an educational program on the responsible conduct of research.

Through this training investigators should understand that approval by the institutional review board is necessary for research on human subjects. Courses should include modules on the special issues related to participation of minorities in clinical research, as well as other subpopulations, including women, children, and vulnerable groups such as the economically disadvantaged, educationally disadvantaged, or the mentally disabled. Many strategies to address the aforementioned barriers can be imparted through such educational activities.

Funders' Roles

Clinical trials can be funded by industry, various entities of the federal government (e.g., National Institutes of Health, Agency for Healthcare Research and Quality, Health Care Financing Administration), state government, and private foundations and organizations. Funders of studies have a responsibility for ensuring that appropriate steps are made to give minorities the opportunity to participate in clinical trials, and because they hold the purse strings they are also in a position to demand strong efforts and ethical principles in recruitment. This responsibility can be imparted to investigators and funded institutions through encouragement, incentives, or requirements for patient recruitment efforts to include attention to minority enrollment. For example, funders can make their decisions to fund a clinical trial based on the track record of institutions or investigators of including minorities in research studies, thereby influencing from the start how investigators design and plan their study regarding subject enrollment. Funders can also require funded investigators and institutions to report on their actual enrollment and efforts taken to recruit minorities.

In cases of large multicenter-collaborative efforts, funders can assist the study teams by developing marketing campaigns that reach appropriate segments of the population. Such large-scale efforts can be designed to reinforce local recruitment efforts of the investigators. It is also important that funders provide the resources to provide participant incentives. Many clinical trial efforts may include provision of an intervention to individuals who have no resources for medical care; or to provide resources to cover the medical care needs of potential participants. For example, a clinical trial comparing different mechanisms of effective community screening for hypertension may need to refer individuals whose blood pressure is not only abnormal, but high enough to demand immediate correction by experienced health professionals. This usually involves making providers accessible and may require providing payment to professionals or institutions to render such care.

In addition, funders should make it financially possible for investigators to provide participant incentives; however, funders need to make sure that such mechanisms do not cause undue pressure for investigators to compromise high ethical standards of involving human subjects in research, including following proper protocols

Table 4. Checklist for Planning and Instituting a Clinical Trial with an Ethnic Minority Population

Personnel trained in ethics and cultural sensitivity	x
Culturally appropriate materials	x
Community liaisons/involvement	x
IRB approval	x
Sufficient funds for incentives	x
Respectful communication throughout the study	x

for obtaining informed consent. All funders, not just the government, should make sure that appropriate approval is sought from the institutional review board, including the procedures for recruitment and retention of individuals.

Summary

Clinical trials are considered to be the most rigorous study design for testing the effects of health and health care interventions. Investigators must be familiar with the historical context of mistrust of the scientific community by ethnic minorities. Recent regulations by the National Institutes of Health may help to increase attention and promote diverse participation in clinical trials. However, knowledge of the barriers affecting participants, investigators, institutions, and funders must all be addressed in attaining full participation. Table 4 provides a practical checklist to use when planning and instituting a clinical trial with an ethnic minority population. Future research should focus on the most effective strategies for enhancing minority participation in clinical trials.

References

Allen M. The dilemma for women of color in clinical trials. *J Am Med Womens Assoc.* 1994;49:105-109.

Angell M. Investigators' Responsibilities for Human Subjects in Developing Countries. *N Engl J Med.* 2000;342:967-969.

Ayanian JZ, et al. The effect of patients' preferences on racial differences in access to renal transplantation. *N Engl J Med.* 1999;341:1661-1669.

Ayanian JZ, et al. Racial differences in the use of revascularization procedures after angiography. *JAMA.* 1993;269:2642-2646.

Ballard E, Nash F, Raiford K, Harrell L. Recruitment of Black Elderly for Clinical Research Studies of Dementia: The CERAD Experience. *Gerontologist.* 1993;33:561-565.

Bennet L. *The Shaping of Black America: The Struggles and Triumphs of African-Americans, 1619 to the 1990s.* Johnson Publishing Company Inc.; 1991.

Blumenthal D, et al. Recruitment and Retention of Subjects for a Longitudinal Study in an Inner-City Black Community. *Health Serv Res.* 1995;30:197-205.

Bowman JE. Tuskegee as a metaphor [letter]. *Science.* 1999;285:47-50.

Brawley OW. The study of untreated syphilis in the negro male [see comments]. *Int J Radiat Oncol Biol Phys.* 1998;40:5-8.

Caplan AL, Annas GJ. Tuskegee as metaphor [letter]. *Science.* 1999;285:48-49.

Carey MP, et al. Reliability and validity of the appraisal of diabetes scale. *J Behav Med.* 1991;14:43-51.

Carrese JA, Rhodes LA. Bridging cultural differences in medical practice. The case of discussing negative information with Navajo patients. *J Gen Intern Med.* 2000;15:92-96.

Carrese JA, Rhodes LA. Western bioethics on the Navajo reservation. Benefit or harm? [see comments]. JAMA. 1995;274:826-829.

Charatz-Litt C. A chronicle of racism: the effects of the white medical community on black health [see comments]. *J Natl Med Assoc*. 1992;84:717-725.

Cooper-Patrick L, et al. Race, gender, and partnership in the patient-physician relationship. JAMA. 1999;282:583-589.

Corbie-Smith G. The continuing legacy of the Tuskegee Syphilis Study: considerations for clinical investigation [see comments]. *Am J Med Sci*. 1999;317:5-8.

Corbie-Smith G. Tuskegee as a metaphor [letter]. *Science*. 1999;285:47-50.

Corbie-Smith G, Thomas SB, Williams MV, Moody-Ayers S. Attitudes and beliefs of African Americans toward participation in medical research. *J Gen Intern Med*. 1999;14:537-546.

Corkery E, et al. Effect of a Bicultural Community Health Worker on Completion of Diabetes Education in a Hispanic Population. *Diabetes Care*. 1996;20:254-257.

Cox JD. Paternalism, informed consent and Tuskegee [editorial; comment]. *Int J Radiat Oncol Biol Phys*. 1998;40:1-2.

Dressler WW. Commentary on "Community Research: Partnership in Black Communities." *Am J Prev Med*. 1993;9:32-34.

el Sadr W, Capps L. The challenge of minority recruitment in clinical trials for AIDS. JAMA. 1992;267:954-957.

Fairchild AL, Bayer R. Uses and abuses of Tuskegee. *Science*. 1999;284:919-921.

Ford E, Cooper R, et al. Coronary arteriography and coronary bypass survey among whites and other racial groups relative to hospital-based incidence rates for coronary artery disease: findings from NHDS. *Am J Public Health*. 1989;79:437-440.

Franks AL, et al. Racial differences in the use of invasive coronary procedures after acute myocardial infarction in Medicare beneficiaries. *Ethnicity Dis*. 1993;3:213-220.

Furth SL, et al. Racial differences in access to the kidney transplant waiting list for children and adolescents with end stage renal disease. *Pediatrics*. 2000;106:756-61.

Gamble VN. A legacy of distrust: African Americans and medical research. *Am J Prev Med*. 1993;9:35-38.

Gamble V. Under the Shadow of Tuskegee: African Americans and Health Care. *Am J Public Health*. 1997;87:1773-1778.

Giles WH, et al. Race and sex differences in rates of invasive cardiac procedures in US hospitals. *Arch Intern Med*. 1995;155:318-324.

Goldberg KC, et al. Racial and community factors influencing coronary artery bypass graft surgery rates for all 1986 Medicare patients. JAMA. 1992;267:1473-1477.

Gorelick PB, Harris Y, Burnett B, Bonecutter FJ. The recruitment triangle: reasons why African Americans enroll, refuse to enroll, or voluntarily withdraw from a clinical trial. An interim report from the African-American Antiplatelet Stroke Prevention Study (AAASPS). *J Natl Med Assoc*. 1998;90:141-145.

Hannan EL, et al. Interracial access to selected cardiac procedures for patients hospitalized with coronary artery disease in New York State. *Med Care*. 1991;29:430-441.

Harris Y, Gorelick PB, Samuels P, Bempong I. Why African Americans may not be participating in clinical trials. *J Natl Med Assoc*. 1996;88:630-634.

Hatch J, et al. Community research: partnership in black communities. *Am J Prev Med*. 1993;9:27-31.

Holder B, et al. Engagement of African American families in research on chronic illness: a multisystem recruitment approach. *Fam Process*. 1998;37:127-151.

Johnson PA, et al. Effect of race on the presentation and management of patients with acute chest pain. *Ann Intern Med*. 1993;118:593-601.

Jones JH. *Bad Blood: The Tuskegee Syphilis Experiment*. New York: The Free Press; 1993.

LaVeist TA, Keith VM, Gutierrez ML. Black/white differences in prenatal care utilization: an assessment of predisposing and enabling factors. *Health Serv Res*. 1995;30:43-58.

Levine DM, Becker DM, Bone LR. Narrowing the gap in health status of minority populations: a community- academic medical center partnership. *Am J Prev Med*. 1992;8:319-323.

Lozano P, Connell FA, Koepsell TD. Use of health services by African American children with asthma on Medicaid. JAMA. 1995;274:469-473.

Lurie P, Wolfe SM. Tuskegee as a metaphor [letter]. *Science*. 1999;285:47-48.

McBean AM, Warren JL, Babish JD. Continuing differences in the rates of percutaneous translu-minal coronary angioplasty and coronary artery bypass graft surgery between elderly black and white Medicare beneficiaries. *Am Heart J.* 1994;127:287-295.

McBride D. Black America: from community health care to crisis medicine [see comments]. *J Health Polit Policy Law.* 1993;18:319-337.

Meinert CL. *Clinical Trials: Design, Conduct, and Analysis.* New York: Oxford University Press; 1986.

Menefee LT. Are black Americans entitled to equal health care? a new research paradigm. *Ethnicity Dis.* 1996;6:56-68.

Millon-Underwood S, Sanders E, Davis M. Determinants of participation in state-of-the-art can-cer prevention, early detection/screening, and treatment trials among African-Americans. *Cancer Nurs.* 1993;16:25-33.

Mirvis DM, et al. Variation in the utilization of cardiac procedures in the Department of Veterans Affairs Health Care System: effect of race. *J Am Coll Cardiologists.* 1994;24:1297-1304.

Moody L, Gregory S, Bocanegra T, Vasey F. Factors Influencing Post-Menopausal African-American Women's Participation in a Clinical Trial. *J Am Acad Nurse Pract.* 1995;7:483-488.

Mouton C, et al. Barriers to Black Women's Participation in Cancer Clinical Trials. *J Natl Med Assoc.* 1997;89:721-727.

NIH Outreach Notebook Committee. Outreach notebook for the NIH guidelines on inclusion of women and minorities as subjects in clinical research. NIH Publication No. 97-4160, 1-35. 1994. National Institutes of Health. Ref Type: Report.

Reynolds PP. The federal government's use of Title VI and Medicare to racially integrate hospi-tals in the United States, 1963 through 1967. *Am J Public Health.* 1997a;87:1850-1858.

Reynolds PP. Hospitals and Civil Rights, 1945-1963: the case of Simkins v Moses H. Cone Memorial Hospital [see comments]. *Ann Intern Med.* 1997b;126:898-906.

Rice MF, Jones W, Jr. Health care, public policy and the courts: black health status as a civil rights issue. *Health Policy.* 1985;5:207-221.

Roberson NL. Clinical trial participation. Viewpoints from racial/ethnic groups. *Cancer.* 1994;74:2687-2691.

Robinson S, Ashley M, Haynes M. Attitudes of African-Americans Regarding Prostate Cancer Clinical Trials. *J Community Health.* 1996;21:77-87.

Roth C, Pinn VW, Bates A, Fanning L. Implementation of the NIH guidelines on the inclusion of women and minorities as subjects in clinical research. Comprehensive Report (Fiscal Year 1997 Tracking Data), 1-19. 1999. Ref Type: Report.

Schulman KA, et al. The effect of race and sex on physicians' recommendations for cardiac catheter-ization [see comments] [published erratum appears in *N Engl J Med.* 1999;340(14):1130]. *N Engl J Med.* 1999;340:618-626.

Shavers-Hornaday VL, et al. Why are African Americans under-represented in medical research studies? Impediments to participation. *Ethnicity Health.* 1997;2:31-45.

Smith DB. Addressing racial inequities in health care: civil rights monitoring and report cards. *J Health Polit Policy Law.* 1998;23:75-105.

Stoy DB, et al. The successful recruitment of elderly black subjects in a clinical trial: the CRISP experience. Cholesterol Reduction in Seniors Program. *J Natl Med Assoc.* 1995;87:280-287.

Suarez L, Lloyd L, Weiss N, Rainbolt T, Pulley L. Effect of social networks on cancer-screening behavior of older Mexican-American women. *J Natl Cancer Inst.* 1994;86:775-779.

Svensson CK. Representation of American blacks in clinical trials of new drugs. *JAMA.* 1989;261:263-265.

Swanson G, Ward A. Recruiting Minorities Into Clinical Trials: Toward a Participant-Friendly System. *J Natl Cancer Inst.* 1995;87:1747-1759.

Talone P. Establishing trust after Tuskegee [editorial]. *Int J Radiat Oncol Biol Phys.* 1998;40:3-4.

Thomas S, Curran J. Tuskegee: From science to conspiracy to metaphor. *Am J Med Sci.*1999;317:1-4.

Thomas S, Quinn S. The Tuskegee Syphilis Study, 1932 to 1972: Implications for HIV Education and AIDS Risk Education Programs in the Black Community. *Am J Public Health.* 1991;81:1498-1504.

Wenneker MB, Epstein AM. Racial inequalities in the use of procedures for patients with ischemic heart disease in Massachusetts. *JAMA.* 1989;261:253-257.

Wermeling D, Selwitz A. Current Issues Surrounding Women and Minorities in Drug Trials. *Ann Pharmacother*. 1993;27:904-911.

Whittle J, Conigliaro J, Good CB, Lofgren RP. Racial differences in the use of invasive cardio-vascular procedures in the Department of Veterans Affairs medical system. *N Engl J Med*. 1993;329:621-627.

Chapter 5

THINKING ABOUT RACE *and* ETHNICITY *in* POPULATION-BASED STUDIES *of* Health

Vickie M. Mays, PhD, MSPH,
Susan D. Cochran, PhD, MS,
and Ninez A. Ponce, PhD, MPP

Introduction

In 1998, President Clinton took a bold step announcing a new initiative aimed at eliminating, by the year 2010, the health disparities long endured by racial and ethnic minority groups in the United States (USDHHS 2000). The president's initiative was driven by a number of factors; among them, several key indicators of the health status of Americans had repeatedly shown disadvantaged health status in racial and ethnic groups when compared to the rest of the population. For example, infant mortality, generally viewed as a problem for developing nations, is estimated as 2.5 times greater for African-Americans in the United States than it is for Whites (Satcher 1999). Despite the fact that the incidence of breast cancer is lower in African-American women than White women, African-American women are more likely to die from it (USDHHS 2000; Mays et al. 2000). Further, African-American men are twice as likely to die from prostate cancer than are White men. Overall, cancer mortality among African-Americans is 30% higher than among Whites (USDHHS 2000).

These health disparities are not limited to Black-White differences. The incidence of cervical cancer is five times greater among Vietnamese women in the United States than it is among White women (Nguyen et al. 2002). Rates of new cases of hepatitis and tuberculosis tend to be higher among Asian and Pacific Islanders living in the United States compared to Whites. Hispanic infants are 1.5 times more likely than White infants to die prematurely (Satcher 1999). The prevalence of dia-

This work was supported in part by the National Institute of Allergy and Infectious Disease (AI 38216), the National Institute of Mental Health (MH 61774), and the National Institute on Drug Abuse (DA 15539). We would like to acknowledge the substantive comments of our colleague Jacqueline Wilson Lucas, MPH, of the National Center for Health Statistics. Statements in this manuscript are the sole responsibility of the authors.

betes in Hispanics, Native Americans, and Alaska Natives is approximately double that seen in Whites (USDHHS 2000). Although Hispanics were only 11% of the population in the United States in 1996, they accounted for nearly 20% of all cases of tuberculosis; they were also twice as likely to die from diabetes and to have higher rates of high blood pressure and obesity than non-Hispanic Whites (USDHHS 2000). Extensive data collected over the last several decades repeatedly show lower life expectancy, higher mortality from cardiovascular disease, lower immunization rates, less access to health insurance coverage, and less intensive health care in some ethnic minority groups when compared to other Americans (National Center for Health Statistics 2000; Institute of Medicine 2002).

Each one of these findings comes from analyses of national population-based survey data such as the National Health Interview Survey. These nationally representative data provide measures of incidence and prevalence of disease, and access to and utilization of medical care, that tend to make the most impact in the federal health policy-setting agenda. We therefore focus our discussion on national, population-based surveys, with a few, though important, references to ongoing state efforts in measuring population-based health.

Considerations in Using Population-Based Samples to Assess Health Issues

Population-based data are used with some confidence in generating reliable estimates of health status, access, and health services utilization of individuals and households. But this degree of certainty is dependent upon researchers having confidence in their knowledge of the size and location of different source populations that comprise American racial/ethnic diversity. Researchers must also be assured that these source populations have been accurately captured and assessed in various data collection procedures.

In the field of public health, studies that use population-based samples are often viewed as a primary source for estimating the incidence and prevalence of health conditions (Rothman and Greenland 1998). Documenting facts about health in different populations also provides a mechanism to measure progress in eliminating health-related inequalities. Without population-based data sets, researchers would be hampered in understanding patterns of disease, including their severity or uniqueness in particular populations, and in determining a need for targeted public health interventions.

At the core of these studies are complicated concerns that intertwine across methodological, social, and public policy issues. Interpreting racial/ethnic data from population-based samples must be done wisely because these findings are used to establish guidelines, design treatments, develop screening criteria, and allocate resources. Population-based samples by the nature of their theoretical basis can falsely lure researchers to statements of certainty, causality, and generalizability about ethnic groups that may be overreaching; those reading and evaluating the results may also give greater weight to study conclusions because of the purported population-based design. Additionally, standard methods in population studies may bias respondent participation in ways that researchers are well aware, but may not fully appreciate. For example, it is widely known that successful recruitment of respondents may depend upon respondent characteristics that can be partially, but not perfectly, adjusted for in later statistical analyses, such as those who have a telephone, whose housing is conventional, whose language of communication is English, or whose jobs are stable.

Issues in Racial and Ethnic Categorizations

There are also other factors that may be well worth considering if the goal is to design and conduct research in a manner that facilitates a better understanding of the contributions of race and ethnicity to health status. The first underlying issue is developing a better understanding of why, how, or whether ethnic or racial categories function as risk indicators for health (Miettinen 1985). Researchers need to grapple with respondent categorizations that permit valid exploration of subgroups' racial and/or ethnic diversity. This is key in determining whether or not observed differences are universal to all ethnic groups, are linked only to specific ethnic subgroups, or are, in actuality, a function of other contextual variables such as neighborhood, social status, or some other explanatory factor (Sue 1999; Buka et al. 2003; Bond Huie, Hummer, and Rogers 2002; Diez-Roux et al. 1997; Anderson et al. 1997). For example, although the National Health Interview Survey (NHIS), an annual household-based survey that interviews respondents from about 45,000 households, has allowed participants to report more than one race since 1976, only recently (data years 1992 through 1996) has the NHIS included racial information by six Asian and three Native Hawaiian and other Pacific Islander groups in its public-use data files (Ponce 1992). Because of this, recent studies could use Asian or Native Hawaiian or other Pacific Islander (NHOPI) subpopulation ethnic group data to demonstrate differences in health status (Kuo 1998) and in patterns of breast cancer and cervical cancer screenings among Asian or NHOPI women (Kagawa-Singer and Pourat 2000). Prior to this study, the normative convention of merging the various Asian and Pacific Islander subgroups into a single category for analytic purposes had the effect of obscuring significant risk variation within this population, making invisible those subgroups at highest risk for late presentation of disease (Kagawa-Singer and Pourat 2000).

While advocating better ethnic or racial categorization as a research goal is relatively easy, doing so methodologically and interpretatively is not. Many have advocated for the use of a "multiple race" categorization in the collection of federal data. As a function of the revised federal race and ethnicity standards issued by the Office of Management and Budget (OMB), Census 2000 allowed respondents to indicate more than one category for their race (OMB 1997a; OMB 1997b; Jones and Smith 2001). But multiple categorization is not necessarily a simple task to accomplish, particularly for states like California or Hawaii that have some of the highest rates of ethnic intermarriage (Jiobu 1988; OMB 1997a; OMB 1997b).

The new federal standards, as currently constructed, allow an individual to check more than one category and direct the federal government in how to collect the data on race and ethnicity. The revised standards have five minimum categories for race:

White, Black/African-American, American Indian/Alaska Natives (AI/AN), Native Hawaiian or other Pacific Islander, and Asian. There are two categories on ethnicity, Hispanic/Latino or non-Latino. Finally, individuals wishing to indicate their mixed racial heritage can select more than one race group to describe themselves. One of the most significant changes was the separation of what was previously the Asian Pacific Islander category into Asian, Native Hawaiians, and other Pacific Islanders.

During the comment period before the directive was established, a number of criticisms emerged. In one instance, a Hawaiian congressional delegation requested the collapse of their racial designation into the American Indian/Alaska Native category. They perceived the AI/AN category as referring to "indigenous people" though this was not the interpretation of the federal government's interagency committee. The view by some ethnic groups of possessing indigenous status can be an important component of their ethnic identity, and these historical roots underscore the complexity of the construct. For example, there are Latino populations, particularly in the Southwest, who are descended from families that have lived in the United States for several generations, some before the establishment of a United States government presence. When asked, they will classify themselves as Native Americans— meaning that they have been in America since before the United States. This classification serves as a way of distinguishing their history from Latinos descended from more recent immigrants. Moreover, many Hispanics do have Indian blood, particularly in California (DiSogra et al. 2002) and so the Native American/American Indian identification reflects true heritage. Yet, we note that in each context, the underlying motivation for claiming the "Native American" identity is very different. Also, the term "native American," when heard in telephone surveys, may elicit affirmative responses among American-born interviewees.

In a nationally representative telephone sample (conducted by Louis Harris and Associates for the Commonwealth Fund on Minority Health (1994)), participants were asked to self-identify as African-American or Black, Hispanic or Latino, non-Hispanic White, Asian, or Native American (Hogue and Hargraves 2000). When data from respondents selecting the "native American" category were examined more closely, many were found to be Hispanic (Mays, Cochran and Sullivan 2000). Use of the census term "American Indian or Alaska Native" would lessen the ambiguity of whether they are Latinos who do have Indian blood, particularly in telephone surveys where there are no visual cues differentiating "Native American" from "native American." More importantly, collection of more detailed information on tribal membership, as is done in the California Health Interview Survey, provides confirmatory information on American Indian or Alaska Native heritage (Satter et al. 2002).

Bridging and Tabulation Methods

With the emergence of more complicated ethnic/racial classification schemes comes a growing body of research indicating differences in health status depending on how an individual's multiple race statuses are tabulated (Mays et al. 2003). Prior to the decennial census, studies were conducted to examine the outcome in coding the combinations of racial and ethnic categories proposed in Census 2000 (OMB 1994; OMB 1995; Baker et al. 1999; Lucas 1999; U.S. Dept. of Labor 1995). Parker (2000) describes three "bridging" approaches (drawn from the OMB)—that is, recategorizing multiple race persons back into a single race group for the purposes of maintaining trends in the data:

- *Deterministic whole assignment*, where multiple race respondents are coded into only one ethnic/racial category. This can be done in several ways including using a "Smallest Group" decision to first assign those reporting both White and any other category to the non-White category, then those reporting two or more non-White categories being assigned to the category with fewest respondents. Conversely, a "Largest Group" approach assigns respondents with two or more racial groups selected to simply the largest group of those selected.

- *Fractional allocation*, in which each multiple race respondent is partially allocated to the relevant groups. How this fraction is determined can vary.

- *Probabilistic allocation*, where a multiple race individual is randomly allocated to a particular group based on some likelihood function.

There are also other possible methods used by states that combine bridging and tabulation approaches. For example, the California Health Interview Survey (CHIS) and other population-based surveys ask for a "primary race identification" among multiracial respondents. This provides deterministic bridging information for those respondents who predominantly identify with one race (Mays et al. 2003). And, for those multiracial individuals not identifying with a single race, a multiple race category could still be tabulated, as it is done in one of the CHIS race tabulations (Ponce 2002). Racial and ethnic tabulation is further complicated with the consideration of treating "Latino/Hispanic origin" as an overlaying ethnicity or as a race. For example, California's Department of Finance tabulates Latino/Hispanic ethnicity as a mutually exclusive race/ethnic category from non-Latino Whites, non-Latino Asians, non-Latino Blacks, non-Latino American Indians, and non-Latino Native Hawaiians and other Pacific Islanders (Mays et al. 2003). The Latino/Hispanic consideration further expands the possibilities of racial and ethnic tabulations and consequent interpretation of health data.

Another approach departs from creating mutually exclusive categories. Baker and colleagues (1999) describe an *"all-inclusive assignment"* where as much information as possible is retained by using one of three codes (only one race classification indicated, one race plus others, or race not indicated) for each ethnic/racial classification for each respondent. With this approach, respondents can appear multiple times and the categories are not mutually exclusive. To illustrate, Baker et al. (1999) presented differences in health profiles using different coding strategies for the parents of respondents in the 1998 Hawaii Health Survey (HHS). This survey is modeled after the National Health Interview Survey, but is conducted as a household telephone survey. Hawaii is a remarkably diverse state with only 67% of the population reporting a single racial background (22% White, 18% Japanese, 13% Filipino, 4% Chinese, 3% Hawaiian, 2% Black). Using the OMB standards for tabulating multiple race data as a starting point, Baker et al. (1999) evaluated ethnic/racial patterns of different health outcomes as a function of two coding permutations (deterministic whole assignment and all-inclusive) with asthma as the health outcome of interest. The effects of these different approaches can be seen in Figures 1-3 using an example of asthma data from the HHS (Baker et al. 1999).

Differences in the racial profile of asthma vary as a function of different bridge method applications. In Figure 1, which shows estimates of asthma prevalence among Whites, the "All-Inclusive" method allocates to "White" anyone reporting any White racial heritage; asthma prevalence is estimated as 9%. In contrast, the "Full" approach includes only those with a single race listed (in this instance, White); by this method asthma prevalence is estimated as 6%. Among multi-race individuals who report being at least partially White (the "Part" classification), prevalence is estimated as 13%. Other race-coding methods generate different outcomes. For example, using a "Smallest Full" approach (those with multiple race backgrounds that include White are allocated fully to the least common race category) drops the prevalence to that of the "Full" classification because multi-race individuals are allocated elsewhere. In contrast, using a "Largest Full" race classification strategy (allocating those with multiple race background to the largest racial category) generates a middle estimate. The "Largest Full" race prevalence is identical to the "All Inclusive" prevalence because Whites are the most common race. In Figure 2, there is less variation in the prevalence of asthma for Hawaiians. But in the final figure (Figure 3) for the Filipino race, the estimated prevalences vary substantially depending on the assignment method employed. Similar variations occurred when prevalence of hypertension was selected as a second health outcome.

To some extent the diversity of Hawaii may seem to overstate the issue; however several states, such as California, Massachusetts, and New York will find themselves struggling with similar decisions (Mays et al. 2003). Findings from national data suggest that changes in health statistics are not limited to racially diverse local-

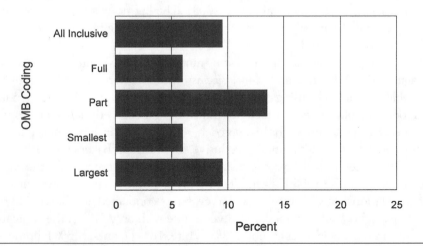

Figure 1. Asthma by OMB Coding—White Race, HHS 1998

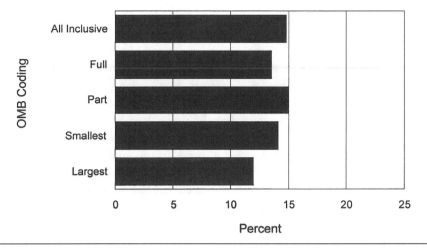

Figure 2. Asthma by OMB Coding—Hawaiian Race, HHS 1998

ities. Data from the 1997 National Health Interview Survey also demonstrate differences in health profiles between single and multiple race tabulations, with American Indian/Alaska Native and White biracial persons having higher smoking rates than either their single race White or single race American Indian/Alaska Native counterparts (Sondik et al. 2000).

Adequacy of Sampling Methods

An important focus of effort for methodologists conducting these surveys is the development of an accurate sampling frame. Some issues are fairly well appreciated, such as whether or not a household has a telephone, but others are more subtle such as fear and community distrust, particularly among ethnic minorities and immigrant

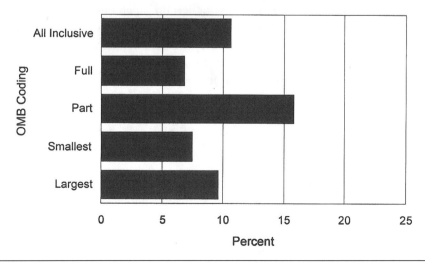

Figure 3. Asthma by OMB Coding—Filipino Race, HHS 1998

populations (Mays 2000). When sampling frames fail to capture the population without bias, then estimates are inaccurate; special efforts by state and local officials for resources, attention, and care of these populations will be necessary in order to advocate for federal funding, policies, and inclusion in the research agenda.

The increasing focus on better specification of health statistics among smaller subpopulations generates a need to consider oversampling strategies to achieve greater statistical power. This is not a new approach, but it does complicate estimation from population-based surveys; in some surveys, even with oversampling, the small numbers of minority participants raise a set of issues in the analyses and interpretation of the data on specific diseases. While multistage probability samples of households used in NCHS studies, such as the NHIS, result in nationally representative data, these samples, though large overall, will at times have insufficient numbers of cases for analyses about diseases that do not occur with high prevalence in a national population—AIDS is one example. Shapiro et al. (1999) estimates, hypothetically, that for a nationally representative survey interviewing approximately 100,000 individuals per year, researchers would need to screen about 1 million persons in an unstratified household sampling to identify 1,000 persons with AIDS. The actual number, though, is probably greater than this because individuals from stigmatized groups or engaging in stigmatized behaviors may for the sake of privacy not acknowledge their disease status during the interview (Shapiro et al. 1999). The ability to find individuals with relatively rare, specific diseases is probably more difficult when the actual number of cases (not the weighted values) are small, which is often the case with ethnic minorities or ethnic minority subgroups.

One major limitation of population-based data is that they are not currently designed to make estimates for small minority groups or to examine ethnic differences within the larger groups. However, these are not insurmountable problems. Sample sizes may be increased to include relevant numbers of particular subpopulations by: 1) collapsing subgroups into an aggregate category to increase sample size—although this may mask critical findings for certain subgroups; 2) combining years of data for analysis, which is something analysts often do—with the tradeoff being the loss of the ability to look at between-year data changes; and 3) oversampling populations—this will increase the costs of surveys and, depending on the method of oversampling, may raise methodological issues on whether and how it can be combined with the random sample, thus complicating the analysis of the data and interpretation of estimates. Despite these tradeoffs, increasing sample sizes to raise the statistical power of estimates for small subpopulation will continue to be important issues for population-based surveys, particularly in light of the call for greater specification of racial/ethnic subgroups.

Targeted surveys that focus specifically on racial/ethnic subgroups is another approach that might ensure that there are sufficient numbers of participants to produce more precise estimates of disease and other health-related information necessary for health planning and health services. For example, the Hispanic Health and Nutrition Examination Survey (Hispanic HANES) conducted by the National Center for Health Statistics used population-based methodology to reach ethnic subpopulations of Hispanics in the United States (USDHHS 1993). Targeted surveys of racial/ethnic groups are still subject to problems of nonresponse and selection bias. But there are some innovative methods for addressing these issues that are worth consideration: Oropesa and Landale (2001) used vital registration systems to design sampling frames in studying maternal-infant health issues in Latino subpopulations, which allowed for the study of nonresponse. In this case, drawing the sample frame from vital registration systems facilitated the identification of the sample along with information on those who chose not to respond.

Setting Health Policy and Health Prevention Agendas

Healthy People 2010 is the Surgeon General's blueprint for disease prevention and health promotion in the U.S. population and will be a principal mechanism for determining the extent to which the President's initiative to eliminate health disparities is accomplished. Achievement of goals established in the document is evaluated by use of quantitative data derived from population-based national health studies, especially those conducted by the National Center for Health Statistics and the Centers for Disease Control and Prevention (Percy and Keppel 2002). Healthy People 2010 contains very broad national health goals for the decade of 2000–2010. Ten leading health indicators will guide the set of targets for Healthy People 2010: physical activity, overweight and obesity, tobacco use, substance abuse, mental health, injury and violence, environmental quality, immunization, responsible sexual behavior, and access to health care. Two themes are dominant throughout: 1) increasing the quality and years of healthy life; and 2) the elimination of racial and ethnic disparities in health status (USDHHS 2000). Most states, governments, and even private funders will use the Healthy People 2010 targets as guidelines for resource allocations for research, prevention, and the setting of policy agendas.

The importance of population-based studies, particularly those under the purview of the federal government, to the prevention agenda of the Healthy People effort seems to have been underscored in recent years when the preparation for Healthy People 2010 was expanded to include more nongovernmental entities and more diverse academic disciplines in the process (USDHHS 2000). The reliance on aggregated population-based studies over convenience samples and clinical data to determine if health targets have been met has generated concerns about the adequacy of national population-based data sources for some minority groups. For example, Asian, Native Hawaiian, and other Pacific Islander community groups pointed to the need for subgroup data as a way of overcoming the phenomenon of obscuring the health status and health needs of subgroups within this community in the comment period for Healthy People 2010. Frontline clinicians and local health care providers complained that they sometimes found themselves faced with a greater occurrence than predicted of some diseases, making it difficult to plan adequately for needed health services. Healthy People 2010 can only be as accurate as the data systems that provide it with information.

Opportunities for measuring important differences across a variety of ethnic groups may be more feasible at the state level and less so at a national level. State-based surveys like the Hawaii Health Survey and the California Health Interview Survey are able to collect data and produce estimates of population characteristics at a more detailed level than is possible with national data (Brown 2001). These datasets impact state policies, but in order to advance the health of specific ethnic groups, they must also be considered as viable sources of population-based data to impact federal priority-setting processes, such as Healthy People 2010.

Census Data Issues

In past years, the census came under fire because of its estimated undercount of 4 million individuals in the 1990 data collection. Apart from its role in reapportionment and redistricting of congressional and state governmental representation, census data also provide the sampling frame of a large number of federally conducted surveys. In addition, census data are used in many studies to produce denominators for various rates and to develop poststratification weights (Botman et al. 2000). Census data also play a primary role in the determination of resource allocation for programs that are often central to the support of the physical, mental, and social health of Americans, particularly the most needy (GAO 1999). Population estimates as derived from census data serve as the primary source for funding allocations by federal, state, and local government, private foundations, and business. The data are central to almost all of the decisions made by federal, state, and local governments

Table 1: Large Formula Grants Programs by Use of Census Data

Formulas That Use Census Data	Estimated Obligations[1]	Percent of Total[2]
Medicaid	104.4	63%
Highway Planning and Construction	19.7	12%
Title 1 Grants to Local Education Agencies	7.5	5%
Foster Care	3.7	2%
Federal Mass Transit Grants	3.1	2%
Community Development Block Grants	3.0	2%
WIC (Food)	3.0	2%
Social Services Block Grant	2.4	1%
Rehabilitation Services: Basic Support	2.2	1%
Employment Training—Dislocated Workers	1.4	1%
Prevention Treatment of Substance Abuse	1.4	1%
HOME Investment Partnerships	1.3	1%
Community Development State Program	1.2	1%
Job Training Partnership Act, Title II-A	1.1	1%
Child Care Development Block Grant	1.0	1%
Vocational Education: Basic Grants	1.0	1%
Job Training Partnership Act, Title II-B	0.9	1%
Adoption Assistance	0.8	0%
Employment Services	0.8	0%
Goals 2000—State and Local Education	0.6	0%
Maternal Child Health Services	0.6	0%
Safe Drug-Free Schools/Communities	0.6	0%
Subtotal	161.6	97%

[1] In billions of dollars.
[2] Rounded to nearest whole number.
GAO, 1999.

in education, public health, transportation, agriculture, and housing. In Table 1, we show federal grant programs that rely on formulas derived from the use of census data (GAO 1999). Several of these programs, such as WIC, Medicaid, and substance abuse prevention programs, are safety-net programs to ensure the health and welfare of some of the neediest Americans. Inaccuracy of census figures can impair health care planning and services in populations that have few other resources.

According to a recent GAO report (1999), the 1990 Census undercount was greatest among African-Americans. Overall, the undercount was higher in large cities, greater for men in comparison to women, and for the young when compared to old (Levine 1991). Latino males, the homeless, and immigrants, particularly new immigrants, were also vulnerable to undercount (Levine 1991). These findings suggest that estimates for large urban areas with underclass populations, such as Texas, New York, Illinois, and California, may have less accuracy and may require researchers to take greater care when conducting analyses and interpreting findings. Bailar (1988), a previous Director of the Census Bureau, has commented that the undercount contributes to obscuring accuracy in our estimates of disease, poverty, unemployment, and crime because the prevalence estimates of these outcomes are benchmarked against the census data to give rate and risk estimates; an example she offers is that of the incidence of AIDS, which is estimated by dividing the number of reported cases by the total number of individuals in a specific population group. If the census substantially undercounts African-American males, their estimated AIDS incidence rate will appear higher than it is in reality.

Critical Data Collection Issues With Racial/Ethnic Minority Populations

In addition to the issues that we have already presented, researchers using population-based samples to assess health status and health behaviors of ethnic minority groups have a number of other concerns with which to contend. In doing so, they will ensure that they can fairly and accurately comment on the population and know how far to generalize their findings.

Male participation. Men's lower participation rate in surveys is a matter that troubles many researchers, but there is a unique set of issues that surrounds the availability and willingness of ethnic minority males to participate in studies (Cochran and Mays 1998). While much has been written about issues of distrust in research participation, there are a number of sampling issues that have unique manifestations in racial/ethnic populations (Mays 2000). Sex ratio imbalance constrains the number of men available for non-institutionalized samples, particularly when the sampling frame is based on households. Ethnic minority men, particularly young African-Americans and Hispanics, are more likely than White men to be in jail, prisons, or other types of incarceration facilities (Mays et al. 2003). Further, urban poor may be less likely to live at a permanent address and as a result may not be counted in household enumeration activities due to their sometimes tenuous residency within the unit. The men, and their health issues, may be underestimated unless there are special efforts to reach them. Adjusting survey weights for nonresponse bias may not solve the difficulty as male respondents who are successfully recruited may differ in important ways from those who are not recruited or choose not to participate.

Institutional vs. noninstitutional sampling frames. The majority of population-based studies are limited to noninstitutionalized populations (the census is an exception as it does count institutionalized persons). As of 2000, approximately 1 million African-Americans were in the prison system (Bonczar and Beck 1997; Palmer 1999). At the current rate of incarceration among African-American males, 1 in 4 (28.5%) is likely to be in prison or jail during his lifetime as compared to 1 in 23 for White males and 1 in 6 for Hispanic males. The likelihood that these men will go to either a state or federal prison varies as a function of age; it is estimated that by the age of 25 years, almost 16% of African-American males, 6% of Hispanics, and 2% of White males will have served some time in state or federal prisons (Bonczar and Beck 1997). Some ethnic minorities, particularly African-Americans and Hispanics, are also more likely to serve in the U.S. military and will be excluded from most sampling frames. Sampling from civilian and non-institutional group living environments, as is done in the National Household Survey on Drug Abuse, still does not capture the homeless or those in residential treatment facilities.

Failure to include respondents outside the normative non-institutionalized sampling frame. This failure has the consequence of differentially harming by race and ethnicity the accuracy of health estimates for some segments of the U.S. population. Because these estimates serve to determine both policy and funding decisions, those population groups that are not well identified may have underserved needs.

Importance of foreign birth and years in the U.S. Population-based health surveys have historically collected information on birth country and number of years of residence in the United States (Loue and Bunce 1999). Studies have indicated that there are different health outcomes for foreign vs. U.S. born subpopulations (Hummer et al. 1999; Singh and Yu 1996; Shiono et al. 1997; King et al. 1999). These may arise from differences in language, diet, habits, values, socioeconomic status, and customs. In addition, measures using the number of years in the United States have served as proxy measures of acculturation (Loue and Bunce 1999). Thus, surveys that collect more detailed information on the temporal nature of the immigrant experience address the heterogeneity of immigrants within racial groups. Studies that simply separate U.S. born from the foreign born may obscure important differences leading to overestimation of risk for one group and underestimation for the other, for example.

Immigration/citizenship status. While indicators of birth country and citizenship status are generally collected in population-based surveys, permanent residency status is often not. Questions on permanent residency status in health surveys can be analyzed to generate estimates of eligibility for particular public health programs such as Medicaid and the Children's Health Insurance Program. Understanding who is and who is not eligible for such services informs public health planners on the needed scope of programs for some uninsured immigrants who would otherwise be marginalized (Loue and Bunce 1999; Ponce et al. 2001). These questions may be considered intrusive to immigrants; a "no" response to a citizenship question may erroneously deem respondents as undocumented immigrants, when in fact these persons could also be legal U.S. entrants with special student or work visas, or could be in the process of permanent residency applications. Fears of deportation may lead to refusals to answer citizenship or birth country questions or discontinuation of survey participation, particularly if the survey is associated with the federal government. Although the questions are intended to track access to health services and health status among immigrants, their sensitive nature has resulted in their omission from many population-based health surveys.

Recent evidence suggests that the questions may be more successful in some state contexts. For example, the California Health Interview Survey, fielded statewide in California in 2001, included a question on whether an immigrant was a permanent resident with a "green card"; the question experienced a very low refusal rate (2%). This may be due in part to two key factors: 1) interviewers stated in the introduction that the research was conducted by a university, and not the government; and 2) the interviewers reiterated confidentiality of respondent identities and that the answers would not be reported to the Immigration and Naturalization Services (Ponce et al. 2003).

Language of interview. Traditionally, most population-based surveys have been conducted in English, and more recently in Spanish as well. Administering an English-only instrument systematically biases a survey's findings to more acculturated immigrant populations who are English proficient. Thus, for example, if a survey was not conducted in Asian languages, then breast cancer screening rates may be biased upward among Asian women, because those who have limited proficiency in English may experience more difficulty in accessing routine health care. Language access is emerging in health policy agendas, catalyzed by the federal government's Culturally and Linguistically Appropriate Services (CLAS) standards for health care, issued in 2000 (Ponce and Penserga 2002). But, when data are not collected from the broader population that includes linguistic minorities, then policies that address the need for language services become difficult, if not impossible, to formulate. Though cost considerations constrain widespread multiple language administration, the number of surveys doing so is growing. Reflecting the linguistic diversity of the population, county and statewide surveys in California, including for example the Los Angeles County Health Survey, the County of Alameda Uninsured Survey, and the California Health Interview Survey, are administered in English, Spanish, and several Asian languages (Ponce et al. 2001; Ponce et al. 2003).

Differential telephone coverage. Several periodic population-based surveys are conducted via telephone including the Behavioral Risk Factor Surveillance System (conducted by the CDC), the National Immunization Survey, and the State and Local Area Integrated Telephone Survey (SLAITS) (the latter two conducted by the National Center for Health Statistics). While ethnic and/or racial differences in telephone coverage are a well-known concern, surveys using telephone methodology have nonetheless proven to be an acceptable method for the collection of data (Weeks et al. 1983; Groves and Kahn, 1979; Yaffe et al. 1978; Hochstim 1967; Aneshensel et al. 1982). It is important to consider, when using data generated by telephone-survey methodology, the quality and nature of the respondents reached. While telephone coverage differences between the various ethnic/racial minority groups and Whites have decreased in recent years, there are still gaps (National Telecommunications and Information Administration 1999). The disparity is more a function of income, as higher income minority households are as likely as White households to have a phone. At the level of incomes of $15,000 and below, however, the disparities are the most pronounced, with only 72% of all American Indians/Eskimos/Aleuts having phones, followed by Blacks at 78%, Whites at 89% and Asian/Pacific Islanders at 91% (National Telecommunications and Information Administration 1999). Overall low-income, young, and specific ethnic groups are less likely than higher income, older Asian/Pacific Islanders to have phones (National Telecommunications and Information Administration 1999). The area with the fewest telephones per household lies in the reservations and trust lands of the Navajo (less than 25%) and Hopi (about 50%) in the American Southwest (American Editor 1998). The states categorized as low in telephone penetration are states with large minority populations (Texas, Illinois, Georgia, Louisiana, South Dakota, Mississippi, Oklahoma, Arkansas, and New Mexico; also Washington, D.C.).

Interviewee's perception of interviewer's race or ethnicity. Another issue to consider in telephone interviews that is often overlooked is the perceived race/ethnicity of the telephone interviewer as determined by vocal cues. Response patterns of ethnic minorities, particularly to sensitive questions involving racial attitudes or areas of racial concern, may be influenced by perceived match or mismatch with the interviewer (Wolford et al. 1995; Kohut 1998). Several studies have found a definite influence of interviewer race on the response of African-Americans to questions concerning racial integration, political attitudes, White hostility, alienation, and other race-related attitudes (Hyman et al. 1954; Schuman and Converse 1971; Campbell 1981; Anderson, Silver and Abramson 1988a,b; Schaeffer 1980; Wolford et al. 1995; Kohut 1998). Historically, surveys began to employ African-American interviewers in response to earlier findings of interviewer-generated effects in order to reduce this bias; however, as noted by Wolford et al. (1995), this practice has decreased in use over time. For example, the later waves of the National Survey of Black Americans and the National Black Election Telephone Panel Study did not use an all-Black interviewing staff as had been done earlier.

Interviewer effects can be quite robust and the direction of bias interjected difficult to predict. Wolford et al. (1995) examined whether race of interviewer might influence the response of African-American participants on race/ethnicity-related items using data from the 1993 National Black Politics Study, which used only Black interviewers, and the National Black Election Study 1984 pre- and postelection interviews. In both surveys, respondents were asked to guess the race of the interviewer, which they did correctly about three-quarters of the time. Wolford et al. (1995) found that when a Black respondent thought the interviewer was White there was a general deference to questions about Whites as well as a warmer attitude toward Whites and White public figures. For those who design population-based telephone surveys in which race/ethnicity related items are included, pretest work to determine the breadth and direction of the bias would be useful (Wolford et al. 1995). Potentially biasing effects can be estimated if a question related to the respondent's perception of the interviewer's race/ethnicity is included in the interview protocol. This seems particularly relevant in studies where researchers are investigating biobehavioral links between health status and social variables such as discrimination, racism, or perceived unfair treatment by Whites (Clark et al. 1999).

Similar issues arise in face-to-face interviews. Often, attempts are made to match the race of interviewer to the race of the household, with the perception that this will minimize any chance of bias as previously discussed. However, the issue of race of interviewers and interviewees is more complicated than it may appear. In a face-to-face interview study of HIV-related risk behaviors of African-American gay men who have sex with men, interviewees were given the choice of the race and sexual orientation of their interviewer. This was done on the basis of focus group results indicating that the men were more comfortable confiding sexual risk-taking behaviors to individuals who were not a part of the Black community and whom they were not likely to encounter in their social networks (Mays and Cochran 1998).

Cultural equivalence. Here in the United States, some researchers attribute health disparities findings across ethnic groups to differences in culturally mediated perceptions of the meaning of the questions that we ask in our studies (Johnson et al. 1996; Andersen, Mullner, and Cornelius 1987; Angel and Thoits 1987; Mays and Cochran 2000; Cochran and Mays 1998; Mays and Jackson 1991). Johnson and colleagues (1996) demonstrated this point in their study assessing differences in social cognition on a set of questions routinely used in health surveys such as the NHIS (global health ratings, disease labeling, health care access, physical activity, depressive symptoms, and nutrition). Using a study population of African-Americans, Mexican Americans, Puerto Ricans, and Whites, they found that even when controlling for variations in education levels there were differences in the perceived meaning of the questions among the various ethnic groups. Some questions even had different perceived meanings between Mexican American and Puerto Rican respondents, despite speaking a common language. For example, a Spanish language survey in Miami found that colloquial or slang terms for concepts differed depending on whether the interviewee was Puerto Rican, Dominican, Haitian, Central American, or a member of another Latino subpopulation.

International health studies recognize the problem of instrument equivalence across populations. Items are viewed as being of either "etic" (culturally general) or "emic" (culturally specific) in their content. Investigators using large-scale population-based data sets with a variety of ethnic group members may want to inquire about any pretest cognitive laboratory work that has been done to establish the "etic" qualities of the questions. Careful interpretation of study findings is also called for when some groups may not be measured as accurately as others.

It is useful to determine whether the issue in question is that of measuring the effects of culture on self-reports of health status or the validity of the questions. An example of this is the recent findings from the Commonwealth study that found that Asians rated their health lower than other ethnic groups (Betancourt, Green, and Carillo 2002). The result may be due to a cultural proscription against answering questions in a way that results in lower status or different interpretation of the given response categories ("excellent," "good," "fair," and "poor"). Each is an issue worthy of consideration in trying to accurately determine the health of racial/ethnic populations.

Aggregated Race Categories

Recognizing who is actually measured in a data set and who is not is tremendously important in interpreting the findings observed in any particular study. In those data sets where the race and ethnic identifier captures only large groups, such as Black/African-American, Hispanic/Latino, Asian/Pacific Islander, and American Indian/Native Alaskan, it may be prudent to consult medical geographers to understand the diversity of the racial/ethnic background of persons captured in the study (Allen and Turner 1988; Allen and Turner 1997). For example, although Southern California is traditionally seen as a gateway for the migration of individuals from Mexico and Central America, it is perhaps less well known that there is also substantial migration to this region from parts of Africa and the West Indies. The effect of this migration pattern on those classified as Black or African-American in the 1990 Census hints at the complicated nature of race and ethnicity in America. Three of the largest Black immigrant groups in Los Angeles are Jamaicans, Belizeans, and Nigerians (Allen and Turner 1997). The Belizian population in Los Angeles is ethnically varied: one subgroup, the Spanish Belizians, came from Belize's northwestern parts that bordered on Mexico and Guatemala; a second group, which is part Mayan Indian, is a mixed Black Caribbean/Indian population known as the Garifunas; and a third subgroup, which is actually the largest of the three, is composed of Creole Belizians. These subgroups can differ in their languages (English, Spanish, or Creole) as well as diet and nutritional habits. These differences might be important to health care planners and providers.

This diversity of people who might be coded with a single aggregated race category in research is not unique to California (Mays et. al 2003) and is a problem often voiced by other states. In southeastern Massachusetts, Cape Verdeans have long been identified as Black despite their heritage as Portuguese. Data from the 1980 Census, for example, indicated that the counties of Chesterfield, South Carolina, Riley, Kansas, and Sweetwater, Wyoming, had high percentages of individuals from East and West Africa.

The Challenges of Contextual Data

Another emerging trend is multilevel studies, where individual-level and group-level factors are simultaneously examined to determine social influences on health (Chen et al. 1998; Krieger et al. 2002; Acevedo-Garcia et al. 2003; Cain 2003; Darity 2003; McLaughlin and Stokes 2002). Including neighborhood characteristics in studies provides new opportunities for environmental epidemiologists to study associations between environmental exposures and the spatial distribution of disease (Massey and Denton 1990 and 1993; Massey, Gross, and Eggers 1991). This mapping of local social characteristics and environmental exposures to individual responses may afford a much better understanding of the health status of ethnic minorities (Baum and Posluszny 1999). Indeed, one of the advantages of multilevel studies is that social level environmental exposures can be directly studied. Ethnic minorities have a high likelihood of experiencing social stressors such as racism, discrimination, and prejudice (Clark et al. 1999; Broman 1996; Mays 1995; Mays and Cochran 1998; Mays, Coleman, and Jackson 1996; Lochner et al. 2001). Multilevel analysis may identify how those exposures work to create health disparities.

In multilevel studies, individual-level data are merged and analyzed with contextual or socioecological data depicting the individual's neighborhood or community, typically defined, because of convenience, by discrete spatial borders such as zip codes, county lines, or metropolitan statistical areas (Diez-Roux 2000). Two main sources of contextual variables in health research are census data and the Area Resource File (ARF). Census data have the advantage of providing socioeconomic characteristics, such as the percent of households living below the poverty level for areas as small as a block-level group, but contain little information on health care. The ARF contains more than 7000 variables with county-level information on health facilities, health professions, measures of resource scarcity, health status, economic activity, health training programs, and other socioeconomic and environmental characteristics. The basic file contains geographic codes and descriptors that enable it to be linked to many other files and to aggregate counties into various geographic groupings. While the ARF has been linked to national population-based surveys, its main disadvantage is that it contains no information for areas smaller than counties.

Newer techniques for capturing "community" and environmental issues focus on "ecologically meaningful" definitions of neighborhoods that may not spatially match census tracts or zip codes. Researchers and even health planners are constructing from individual-level surveys, group-level measures of social cohesion, trust and reciprocated exchange that impact health status (Earls and Buka 1997). A growing body of research has demonstrated that group-level measures of the degree of social cohesion in a neighborhood may be related to the promotion of healthy behaviors. This neighborhood-level effect may have a bigger impact in racial/ethnic minority populations. Indeed, Buka et al. (2003) have shown that the degree of a neighborhood's social cohesion significantly increased the odds of a higher birthweight among African-American babies, but not among White babies (Buka et al. 2003). Inclusion of contextual measures should be considered for population-based health surveys in that many of the "unmeasured" factors involved in ethnic and racial health disparities may arise from intrinsic social disparities across communities.

Summary

In this chapter we have focused on some of the challenges that researchers and policy makers face in the use of national population-based datasets when they seek to determine and monitor the health of racial and ethnic minority groups in the United States. These challenges include making decisions about the classification of race and ethnicity, developing sampling designs that address problems in participation by racial/ethnic minority males and creating survey instruments that capture the influences of immigrant status and language variations, collecting information from respondents in culturally competent context, and merging contextual data to population-based datasets. Despite the challenges that exist in using national population-based datasets, they nonetheless continue to be an important resource for health investigations of racial and ethnic minority groups. Our hope is that methodologies are developed that contribute to achieving the Healthy People 2010 goal of eliminating health disparities in racial/ethnic populations in the United States.

References

Acevedo-Garcia D, Lochner KA, Osypuk TL, Subramanian SV. Future directions in residential segregation and health research: a multi-level approach. *Am J Public Health.* 2003;93:215-225.

Allen J P, Turner EJ. *The ethnic quilt—population diversity in Southern California.* Northridge, CA: The Center for Geographical Studies: California State University, Northridge; 1997.

Allen JP, Turner EJ. *We the People: An Atlas of America's Ethnic Diversity.* New York: MacMillan; 1988.

American Editor. Minorities, information, technologies and libraries. July–August 1998. Available at: http://www.libraries.psu.edu/divers/conf/minority.htm.

Andersen RN, Mullner RM, Cornelius, LJ. Black white differences in health status: Methods of substance. *Milbank Q.*1987;65(suppl 1):72-99.

Anderson B, Silver BD, Abramson PR. The effects of race of the interviewer on measures of electoral participation by Blacks in SRC National Election Studies. *Public Opinion Q.* 1988a; 52(1):53-83.

Anderson B, Silver BD, Abramson PR. The effects of race of the interviewer on race related attitudes of Black respondents in SRC/CPS national election studies. *Public Opinion Q.* 1988b; 52(3):289-324.

Anderson RT, Sorlie P, et al. Mortality effects of community socioeconomic status. *Epidemiology.* 1997;8(1):42-7.

Aneshensel CS, Frerichs RR, Clark VA, Yokopenic PA. Measuring depression in the community: A comparison of telephone and personal interviews. *Public Opinion Q.* 1982;46:110-121.

Angel R, Thoits P. The impact of culture on the cognitive structure of illness. *Culture Med Psychiatry.* 1987;11:465-494.

Bailar B. The miscounting of America. *Washington Post.* March 6, 1988:pC3.

Baker KK, Onaka AT, Reyes-Salvail F, Horiuchi B, Dannemiller J, Tom T, Zhang J, Tanaka C. Multi-race health statistics: A state perspective Hawaii Health Survey (HHS). *Proceedings of the 1999 National Conference on Health Statistics.* Washington, D.C. (PHS) 00-1025, 1999.

Baum A, Posluszny DM. Health Psychology: Mapping biobehavioral contributions to health and illness. *Ann Rev Psychol.* 1999;50:137-163.

Betancourt JR, Green AR, & Carillo JE. Cultural competence in health care: Emerging frameworks and practical approaches. The Commonwealth Fund. 2002; 576. Available at: http://www.cmwf.org/programs/minority/betancourt_culturalcompetence_576.pdf.

Bonczar TP, Beck AJ. *Lifetime likelihood of going to a state or federal prison.* Bureau of Justice Statistics Special Report, NCJ-160092, 1997

Bond Huie SA, Hummer RA, Rogers RG. Individual and contextual risks of death among race and ethnic groups in the United States. *J Health Soc Behav.* 2002;43(3):359-381.

Botman SL, Moore TF, Moriarity CL, Parsons VL. Design and estimation for the National Health Interview Survey, 1995-2004. *NCHS Vital Health Stat.* 2000;2(130).

Browman CL. The health consequences of racial discrimination: A study of African-Americans. *Ethnicity Dis.* 1996;6:148-153.

Brown, ER. Science and Politics in Meeting Policy Needs for Population Health Assessment in the Most Diverse State. 129th Annual American Public Health Association Meeting. October 29, 2001. Available at: http://www.apha.org/meetings/future_past.htm.

Buka SL, Brennan RT, Rich-Edward JW, Raudenbusch SW, Earls F. Neighborhood support and the birth weight of urban infants. *Am J Epidemiol.* 2003;157:1-8.

Cain VS. Investigating the role of racial/ethnic bias in health outcomes. *Am J Public Health*. 2003; 93:191-195.

Campbell A. *The sense of well-being in America*. New York: McGraw-Hill; 1981.

Chen FM, Breiman RF, Farley M, Plikaytis B, Deaver K, Cetron MS. Geocoding and linking data from population-based surveillance and the US Census to evaluate the impact of median household income on the epidemiology of invasive Streptococcus pneumoniae infections. *Am J Epidemiol*. 1998;148:1212-1218.

Clark R, Anderson NB, Clark V, Williams DR. Racism as a stressor for African-Americans: A Biopsychosocial model. *Am Psychol*. 1999;54:805-816.

Cochran SD, Mays VM. Use of a telephone interview survey to assess HIV risk among African-American and Hispanic Los Angeles County residents. *Proceedings of the 27th Public Health Conference on Records and Statistics and the National Committee on Vital and Health Statistics 47th Annual Symposium*. Washington, D.C.: USDHHS; 1998.

Darity WA. Employment discrimination, segregation, and health. *Am J Public Health*. 2003;93:226-231.

Diez-Roux AV. Multilevel analysis in public health research. *Ann Rev Public Health*. 2000;21:171-192.

Diez-Roux AV, Nieto FJ, et al. Neighborhood environments and coronary heart disease: a multilevel analysis. *Am J Epidemiol*. 1997;146:48-63.

DiSogra C, Ponce NA, Yen W, Brown, ER, Satter DE. Creating a single race/ethnicity variable for the highly diverse sample in the 2001 California Health Interview Survey, 130th Annual Meeting of the American Public Health Association, Nov. 11, 2002. Available at: http://www.apha.org/meetings/future_past.htm.

Earls F, Buka SL. *Project on human development in Chicago neighborhoods*. Washington, D.C.: National Institute of Justice; 1997.

Government Accounting Office. *Formula Grants: Effects of Adjusted Population Counts on federal funding to states*. Washington, D.C.: U.S. Health, Education and Human Service Division, U.S. Government Printing Office, GAO/HEHS-99-69; 1999.

Groves RM, Kahn RL. *Surveys by Telephone: A National Comparison with Personal Interviews*. New York: Academic Press; 1979.

Hochstim JR. A critical comparison of three strategies of collecting data from households. *Journal of the American Statistical Association*. 1967;62:976-989.

Hogue C, Hargraves MA. The Commonwealth Minority Fund of 1994: An overview. In: Hogue C, Hargraves MA, Scott KS, eds. *Minority Health in America: Findings and policy implications from the Commonwealth Fund Minority Health Survey*. Baltimore: John Hopkins Press; 2000.

Hummer RA, Rogers RG, Nam CB, LeClere FB. Race/ethnicity, nativity, and U.S, adult mortality. *Soc Sci Q*. 1999;80:136-153.

Hyman HH, Cobb WJ, Feldman JJ, Hart CW, Stember CH. *Interviewing in Social Research*. Chicago: University of Chicago Press; 1954.

Institute of Medicine (IOM). *Care Without Coverage: Too Little, Too Late*. (Committee on the Consequences of Uninsurance, Board on Health Care Services). Washington D.C.: National Academy Press; 2002.

Jiobu RM. *Ethnicity and Assimilation: Blacks, Chinese, Filipinos, Japanese, Koreans, Mexicans, Vietnamese, and Whites*. Buffalo, N.Y.: SUNY University Press; 1988.

Johnson TP, O'Rourke D, Chavez N, Sudman S, Warnecke RB, Lacey L, Horm J. Cultural variations in the interpretation of health survey questions. In: Warnecke R, ed. *Health survey research methods: Conference Proceedings*. Hyattsville, MD: USDHHS, PHS (PHS 96-1013), 1996:57-62.

Jones NA, Smith AS. The two or more races population: 2000. Census 2000 Brief. U.S. Department of Commerce, Economics and Statistics Administration. Washington, D.C.; 2001

Kagawa-Singer M, Pourat N. Asian American and Pacific Islander breast and cervical carcinoma screening rates and healthy people 2000 objectives. *Cancer*. 2000;89:696-705.

King G, Polendak AP, Bendel R, Hovey D. Cigarette snoking among native and foreign-born African-Americans. *Ann Epidemiol*. 1999;9:236-244.

Kohut A. Bias in the polls: It's not political, it's racial: Pew Research Center Biennial News Consumption Survey. *American Editor*. (July 1998). Available at: http://www.asne.org/kiosk/editor/98.july/kohut1.htm.

Krieger N, Chen JT, Waterman PD, Soobader M-J, Subramanian SV, Carson R. Geocoding and monitoring US socioeconomic inequalities in mortality and cancer incidence: does choice of area-based measure and geographic level matter? The Public Health Disparities Geocoding Project. Am J Epidemiol. 2002;156:471-482

Kuo J. Health status of Asian Americans: United States 1992-1994. Advance data from vital and health statistics; no. 298. Hyattsville, Md.: National Center for Health Statistics; 1998.

Levine R. Census adjustment means more for New York (1990 undercount adjustment survey's impact on Metropolitan New York City). New York Times. June 14 1991:pB7(L).

Lochner K, Pamuk E, Makuc D, Kennedy BP, Kawachi I. State-level income inequality and individual mortality risk: A prospective, multilevel study. Am J Public Health. 2001;91:385-391.

Loue S, Bunce A. The Assessment of Immigration Status in Health Research No. 127. Draft Version. The Assessment of Immigration Status in Health Research. (PHS) 99-1327; 1999.

Lucas JW. Crossing New Frontiers: National Health Interview Survey Race and Ethnicity Data Revisited. Proceedings of the 1999 National Conference on Health Statistics. Washington, D.C.: (PHS) 00-1025. 1999.

Massey DS, Denton NA. American apartheid: Segregation and the making of the underclass. Am J Sociology. 1990;76:329-357.

Massey DS, Denton NA. American apartheid: Segregation and the making of the underclass. Cambridge, Mass.: Harvard University Press;1993.

Massey DS, Gross AB, Eggers ML. Segregation, the concentration of poverty and the life chances of individuals. Soc Sci Res. 1991;20:397-420.

Mays VM. Black women, work, stress, and perceived discrimination: The Focused Support Group Model as an intervention for stress reduction. Cultural Diversity Ment Health. 1995;1:53-65.

Mays VM. Methods for increasing recruitment and retention of ethnic minorities in health research through addressing ethical concerns. In Cynamon ML, Kulka RA, eds. Proceedings of the Seventh Conference on Health Survey Research Methodology. Washington, D.C.: National Center for Health Statistics, USDHHS (PHS) 01-1013; 2000. Available at: http://www.cdc.gov/nchs/data/conf/conf07.pdf.

Mays VM, Cochran SD. Racial discrimination and health outcomes in African-Americans. Proceedings of the 27th Public Health Conference on Records and Statistics and the National Committee on Vital and Health Statistics 47th Annual Symposium. Washington, D.C.: USDHHS. 1998.

Mays VM, Cochran SD. Methods for increasing the relevance of telephone and field survey research to community needs. Proceedings of the National Center for Health Statistics Conference on National Health Statistics. Aug. 2-4, 1999. Washington, D.C.: USDHHS. 2000.

Mays VM, Cochran SD, Sullivan JS. Health care for African-American and Hispanic women: Report on perceived health status, access to care and utilization patterns. In C. Hogue, M.A. Hargraves, KS Scott, eds. Minority Health in America: Findings and policy implications from the Commonwealth Fund Minority Health Survey. Baltimore: John Hopkins Press; 2000.

Mays VM, Coleman LM, Jackson JS. Perceived race-based discrimination, employment status, and job stress in a national sample of Black women: Implications for health outcomes. J Occup Health Psychol. 1996;1:319-329.

Mays VM, Jackson JS. AIDS survey methodology with Black Americans. Soc Sci Med. 1991;33:47-54.

Mays VM, Million-Underwood S, Phillips J, Guidry JJ, Matthews-Juarez P. Psychosocial/ Behavioral Issues in breast cancer prevention, control, treatment and research. Paper presented at: African-American Research Summit on Breast Cancer, Washington, D.C., Sept. 8-10, 2000.

Mays VM, Ponce NA, Washington DL, Cochran SD. Classification of race and ethnicity: Implications for public health. Ann Rev Public Health. 2003;24:83-110. Available at: http://publhealth. annualreviews.org/cgi/content/full/24/1/83?ijkey=5G395NlxSzz5okeytype=refsiteid=arjournals.

McLaughlin DK, Stokes SC. Income inequality and mortality in US counties: Does minority racial concentration matter? Am J Public Health. 2002;92:99-105.

Miettinen OS. Theoretical Epidemiology. New York: John Wiley; 1985.

National Center for Health Statistics. Health, United States, 2000 with Adolescent Health Chartbook. Hyattsville, Md.: National Center for Health Statistics; 2000.

National Telecommunications and Information Administration. *Falling through the net: Defining the digital divide*. Technical report, US Department of Commerce, 1999. Available at: http://www.ntia.doc.gov/ntiahome/fttn99/FTTN.pdf

Nguyen TT, McPhee SJ, Nguyen T, Lam T, Mock J. Predictors of cervical Pap Smear screening awareness, intention, and receipt among Vietnamese-American women. *Am J Preventative Med*. 2002;23:207-214.

Office of Management and Budget (OMB). *Recommendations from the Interagency Committee for the Review of the Racial and Ethnic Standards to the Office of Management and Budget Concerning Changes to the Standards for the Classification of Federal Data on Race and Ethnicity*. Federal Register 1997a;62(131):36874-36946.

Office of Management and Budget (OMB). *Revisions to the Standards for the Classification of Federal Data on Race and Ethnicity*. Federal Register 1997b;62(210):58782-58790.

Office of Management and Budget (OMB). *Standards for the classification of federal data on race and ethnicity*. Federal Register, 1995;60(166)(60FR44674-93):29831-29835.

Office of Management and Budget (OMB). *Standards for the classification of federal data on race and ethnicity*. Federal Register, 1994;59(123)(59FR29831-35):29831-29835.

Oropesa RS, Landale NS. Nonresponse in maternal-infant health surveys of "rare" and "not-so-rare" Latino populations: Findings from a study of Mainland and Island Puerto Ricans. Working Paper 01-06. University Park, Pa.: Population Research Institute, Pennsylvania State University. 2001.

Palmer LS. Number of Blacks in prison nears 1 million. *Boston Globe/Seattle Post-Intelligencer*. March 2, 1999. Available at: http://www.hemp.net/news/9903/05/million_blacks_in_prison.html.

Parker JD. Bridge methods for comparing race-specific data collected before and after implementation of the revised OMB standard. *Proceedings of the National Center for Health Statistics Conference on National Health Statistics*. (Aug 2-4, 1999). Washington, D.C.: USDHHS; 2000.

Percy JN, Keppel KG. A summary measure of health disparity. *Public Health Rep*. 2002;117: 273-280.

Ponce NA. A research plan to advance the understanding of the health of Asians and Pacific Islanders—NCHS Initiative. 1992. Available at: http://www.cdc.gov/nchs/otheract/grants/projects/progdir/ponce.htm

Ponce NA. The California Health Interview Survey: Measuring multi-racial health: counts, rates and artifacts. Paper presented at: California Pan Ethnic Health Network, Oakland, Calif., Oct. 22, 2002. Available at: http://www.cpehn.org/html/whatsnew.html.

Ponce NA, Conner T, Barrera P, Suh D. Advancing Universal Coverage in Alameda County. Los Angeles: UCLA Center for Health Policy Research Summary Report. 2001.

Ponce NA, Lavarreda SA, Yen W, Satter D, DiSogra C, Brown ER. The California Health Interview Survey: translation methodology of a major survey for California's multi-ethnic population. Manuscript under review; 2003.

Ponce NA, Penserga L. Language Access in Health Care: Why the Policy and Practice Inertia? *Harvard Health Policy Rev*. Fall 2002;3:1-2.

Rothman KJ, Greenland S. *Modern Epidemiology*, 2nd Edition. Philadelphia: Lippincott–Raven; 1998.

Satter, DE, Mader SJ, Sen R, Keeler C, Yen W, DiSogra C, Brown ER. Surveying the Health Needs of American Indian and Alaska Natives (AIAN)—The California Health Interview Survey 2001 and Its AIAN Oversample. 130th Annual Meting of the American Public Health Association, Nov. 11, 2002. Available at: http://www.apha.org/meetings/ future_past.htm.

Satcher DS. Healthy People at 2010. *Public Health Rep*. 1999;114:563.

Schaeffer NC. Evaluating race-of -interviewer effects in a national survey. *Soc Methods Res*. 1980; 8:400-419.

Shapiro MF, Berk ML, Berry SH, Emmons CA, Athey LA, Hsia DC, Leibowitz AA, Maida CA, Marcus M, Perlman JF, Schur CL, Schuster MA, Senterfitt JW, Bozzette SA. National probability samples in studies of low-prevalence diseases. Part I: Perspectives and lessons from the HIV cost and services utilization study. *Health Services Res*. 1999;34(5 Pt 1):951-968.

Shuman H, Converse J. The effects of Black and White interviewers on Black responses. *Public Opinion Q*. 1971;35:1.

Shiono PH, Rauh VA, Park M, Lederma SA, Zuskar D. Ethnic differences in birthweight: the role of lifestyle and other factors. *Am J Public Health*. 1997;87:787-793.

Singh GK, Yu SM. Adverse pregnancy outcomes: differences between U.S. and foreign-born women in major US racial and ethnic groups. *Am J Public Health.* 1996;86:837-843.

Sondik EJ, Lucas JW, Madans JH, Smith SS. Race/ethnicity and the 2000 census: Implications for public health. *Am J Public Health.* 2000;90:1709-1713.

Sue S. Science, ethnicity and bias: Where have we gone wrong? *Am Psychol,* 1999;54:1070-1077.

United States Census Bureau. The Foreign-Born Population in the United States: March 1999. *Current Population Reports, Population Characteristics,* Series P20-519; 2000.

United States Department of Health and Human Services. National Center for Health Statistics. HISPANIC Health and Nutrition Examination Survey, 1982–1984 [Computer file]. 8th release. Hyattsville, Md.: U.S. Dept of Health and Human Services, National Center for Health Statistics [producer], 1992. Ann Arbor, Mich.: Inter-university Consortium for Political and Social Research [distributor]; 1993.

United States Department of Health and Human Services. Healthy People 2010. Available at: http://www.health.gov/healthypeople/Document/html/volume1/goal.html; 2000.

United States Department of Labor. *A CPS supplement for testing methods of collecting racial and ethnic information: May 1995.* Bureau of Labor Statistics; 1995. Available at: http:// stats.bls.gov/ news.release/ethnic.toc.htm.

Weeks MF, Kulka RA, Lessler JT, Whitmore RW. Personal versus telephone surveys for collecting household health data at the local level. *Am J Public Health.* 1983;73:1389-1394.

Wolford ML, Brown RE, Marsden A, Jackson JS, Harrison C. Bias in telephone surveys of African-Americans: The impact of perceived race of interviewer on responses. *Proceedings of the Section on Survey Research Methods,* American Statistical Association; Aug. 13-17, 1995. Available at: http://www.amstat.org/sections/srms/proceedings/y1995f.html.

Yaffe R, Shapiro S, Fuchsberg RR, Rohde CA, Corpeno HC. Medical Economics Survey-Methods Study: Cost effectiveness of alternative survey strategies. *Med Care.* 1978;16:641-659.

Chapter 6

BEHAVIORAL STUDIES

Deborah Parra-Medina, PhD, MPH,
and Elizabeth Fore, MEd

Introduction

In recent years, national health agencies have sounded a call for research and interventions to reduce or eliminate the persistent racial and ethnic disparities in health indicators—disparities that they acknowledge are clearly linked to inequalities in income and education (USDHHS 2000; National Institutes of Health 2000). There is a growing recognition among scholars that bio-medical and individualized behavioral approaches to health research and health interventions have failed to reduce disparities (Orleans et al. 1999; Wallack 2000; Emmons 2000); a change in research methodology is needed to investigate and eliminate these health disparities. The following chapter suggests some reasons why previous approaches may not have been effective in closing the gap in health status among different groups of people and provides recommendations for research focused on redressing those limitations to create interventions that are more effective and produce a more equitable and healthy society.

Until the early 1980s, race/ethnicity, culture, and other dimensions of social difference were largely ignored in health behavior theories, and interventions were modeled on those theories (Becker 1974). These early theories were developed to explain individual health behavior and ignored external forces that could influence or shape an individual's health behaviors. The prevailing theories assumed that individuals had the ultimate control over their health behaviors and thus the responsibility for their health. Continued dependence on interventions that emphasize intrapersonal theories of health and that ignore the social, political, and economic environments are unlikely to eliminate public health disparities centered on race/ethnic, socioeconomic, gender, and other dimensions of social inequality.

Individual Models of Health

Four of the most widely used health behavior change theories address only intra-personal and interpersonal aspects of health behavior and overlook cultural, social, political, and economic influences and barriers; as a result, behavioral change interventions based on these theories tend to be focused at the individual level only. Interventions targeting changes in the cultural, social, and political environment are not addressed. The Health Belief Model (Becker 1974; Janz and Becker 1984; Rosenstock 1966; Rosenstock 1974), Social Cognitive Theory (Bandura 1991; Bandura 1989; Bandura 1986), the Theory of Reasoned Action (Ajzen and Fishbein 1980; Fishbein 1980; Fishbein 1975), and the Transtheoretical Model (Prochaska and DiClemente 1983) are inadequate in their ability to generalize across racial/ethnic, social, economic, and cultural lines because of their limitations in addressing environmental causes of poor health and barriers to the adoption of positive health behaviors. The fact that these theories have been deemed relevant to the health of racial/ethnic minorities, women, and the poor is related more to their popularity among health psychologists and public health educators in the United States than to their proven relevance to these groups of people (Elder et al. 1998).

The Health Belief Model (HBM) was initially formulated to help explain why people did not participate in programs to detect or prevent disease (Rosenstock 1966; Rosenstock 1974) and was later extended to examine behavior in response to diagnosed illness (Becker 1974). The HBM has been characterized as a value-expectancy model because it encompasses the desire to get well or to avoid illness (value) and the belief that a specific action will help the person prevent or alleviate illness symptoms (expectations). Developers of the HBM maintain that health-related behaviors are determined by whether individuals (a) perceive themselves to be susceptible to a particular health problem; (b) see this problem as a serious one; (c) are convinced that treatment or prevention activities are effective yet not overly costly in terms of money, effort, or pain; and (d) are exposed to a prompt or cue to take health action.

In contrast to the Health Belief Model, the Theory of Reasoned Action addresses both intrapersonal and interpersonal influences on behavior change. The Theory of Reasoned Action places relatively more emphasis on the concept of "behavioral intention," which in turn can be predicted by the person's expectations and attitudes regarding the outcomes of a behavior, and his/her normative beliefs with respect to what "influentials" (especially peers) would do in a specific situation. This theory presupposes that most socially relevant behaviors are voluntary, and may be effected either by attitude or behavior (Ajzen and Fishbein 1980).

Although Ajzen and Fishbein (1980) address the impact of peer influence on an individual's behavior, Social Cognitive Theory (SCT) takes a broader look at outside influences. Social Cognitive Theory emphasizes the interaction between a person's mental processes (especially knowledge, attitudes, and emotions) and his/her environment and behavior. In this model, the environment is defined as external factors that affect the individual. The constructs of person, environment, and behavior interact dynamically in a process called "reciprocal determinism." The social cognitive emphasis is on the concepts of outcome expectations and self-efficacy. Outcome expectations that overlap substantially with parallel concepts in the Theory of Reasoned Action and the Heath Belief Model represent the expectation that a positive outcome or consequence will occur as a function of the behavior. Self-efficacy is a person's perception that he or she has the appropriate skills and is capable of performing a specific behavior (Bandura 1989). Although Social Cognitive Theory addresses environmental barriers to the adoption of positive health behaviors, this model is directed at the individual-level. Rather than targeting change to a hostile environment, interventions are focused on helping the individual to develop the skills to change his/her behavior despite antagonistic external influences.

Another widely used theory that does include a limited emphasis on external factors is the Transtheoretical Model (TTM) or Stages of Change, which has been applied to a variety of recent health promotion efforts, including in the areas of smoking cessation, promotion of cancer screening, and, recently, smoking prevention. According to Prochaska and DiClemente (1983), behavior change progresses from a person being in the precontemplation stage (not even thinking about changing a specific behavior) to the contemplation phase (starting to consider but not yet actually acting on a behavior change course), to the action stage (making the initial steps toward behavior change, to the maintenance stage (maintaining behavior change and not even thinking about going back). Although outside influences such as policies or social support may influence or inhibit behavior, the theory rests on individual psychological change and interventions are planned for the individual. With few exceptions policy or societal changes are not the foci of interventions using the TTM (Auslander et al. 2000).

Although these theories and models have been used extensively in health promotion programs, they ignore the context of an individual's life. The individual is the starting point of the theory and the unit of analysis in this research. Emphasis is placed on primary prevention and individual responsibility for producing and maintaining health. The social environment is viewed as affecting health but the focus is on making positive choices to enhance one's own health; there is an unspoken assumption that with the right motivation and with the opportunities to pursue healthful activities, people will want to do so (Ruzek 1997). Some would argue that society, not individuals, should be viewed as responsible for creating the social conditions that produce health damaging behaviors that health promoters purportedly see only as characteristics of individuals (Ruzek 1997).

Addressing the environmental context of an individual's life is essential in promoting better health for the whole community, but the contributions made by individual approaches to behavior change should not be discounted. The Robert Wood Johnson Foundation recently conducted an assessment of progress in population-based health promotion in six areas of behavioral health (tobacco use, alcohol abuse, drug abuse, unhealthy diet, sedentary lifestyle, and risky sexual practices), and concluded that more progress has been made in developing and implementing individually oriented interventions than in developing and implementing environmentally-focused interventions, even though the latter are necessary for greatest population impact (Orleans et al. 1999). The researchers conclude that at the individual level, there are reasonably effective interventions for these six risk factors, but individual-level approaches are limited in their potential for health behavior change if they are conducted in isolation without the benefit of interventions and policies that also address interpersonal and societal factors that influence health behaviors.

Discrimination, policies, family, culture, and organizations can all facilitate or inhibit positive health behaviors (Council of Scientific Affairs 1991; Masi et al. 1995). Because they emerged from the study of dominant-culture middle-class populations, existing models and analyses can only provide limited explanatory power if applied directly to poor or racial/ethnic groups. The role of societal factors in determining health was not seen as a problem in the past because the individuals doing the research were male scholars for whom the macro social structures are a support, not an impediment to health.

The failure of individual models of health behavior change to explain and to reduce persistent and pervasive health disparities across race, class, gender, sexuality, and other dimensions of inequality results from the way that these dimensions are treated in most health research—as control variables in quantitative analyses that go undefined and unanalyzed (Loue 1999; Rivara and Finberg 2001; Williams 1997; Senior and Bhopal 1994). Health researchers continue to report findings on the basis of race, class, and gender without an in-depth exploration of what observed associations may signify (Williams and Collins 1995; LaVeist 1994). Some work does attempt to decipher the meaning of these variables and their connections to health and illness by looking for intervening factors to explain their effects on a particular health outcome. For example, some common intervening factors in mental health research on depression in women include sense of control, resilience, stress, role overload, and social supports (Weber, Hancock, and Higginbotham 1997). But, even when these factors reduce or explain the variance in particular depression indicators attributed to race, gender, class, or socioeconomic status, they still leave fundamental questions about how these systems of inequality operate in individual lives and group processes (i.e., their mechanisms, how they are experienced). We remain unclear about how they shape mental health and what can be done to improve health outcomes through behavioral interventions.

Those questions linger in part because the individual is the primary focus of attention in most health research paradigms; by focusing on the individual and structuring research accordingly; however, we cannot address the fundamental character of race, social class, and gender that take meaning in social groups. These individual characteristics are social constructs, defined by historical, geographic, and cultural context, and are not immutable or biologically determined. Consequently, when for purposes of research we designate an *individual* as of a particular race or gender, for example, we have merely given ourselves a static marker of *the place to go* if we actually want to observe and to understand how those systemic group processes produce social inequality and shape health outcomes. The first step in eliminating health disparities across race/ethnicity, social class, and gender is the delineation within our research of what these systems of social inequality are: how they are constructed, how they are reproduced, how they change, and how they intersect with one another and with health.

Understanding Social Inequalities in Health

Individual health models lack a conceptual framework that allows for the identification of social processes that shape disparities. In her book, *Understanding Race, Class, Gender, and Sexuality*, Lynn Weber (Weber 2001) presents a conceptual framework that she derived by exploring common themes that have characterized approximately 20 years of feminist scholarship seeking to understand the intersecting dynamics of race, class, gender, sexuality, and other dimensions of inequality. The themes presented by Weber allow for the identification of underlying structural mechanisms that shape health disparities and suggest questions and methods to aid in the search for the connections between race, class, gender, and sexuality and health.

Understanding these disparities requires further research into the broader social, cultural, economic, and political processes that influence the nature and extent of disparities (House and Williams 2000). The themes of Weber's (Weber 2001) framework explore race, class, gender, and sexuality as social systems—patterns of social relationships among people—that are:

complex	intricate and interconnected
pervasive	widespread throughout all societal domains, e.g., in families and communities, in health, religion, education, the economy, government, the law and criminal justice, the media
dynamic	changing, always transforming
persistent	prevailing over time and across places
severe	serious in their consequences for social life
hierarchical	unequal, stratified (ranked), benefiting and providing options and resources for some by harming and restricting options and resources for others.

According to Weber (Weber 2001), race, class, gender, and sexuality can be conceptualized as systems of inequality that can only be understood in their historical and global/geographic context; therefore, research should focus on specific times and places and avoid the search for universal truths. These systems are socially constructed, not biologically determined. Their meaning develops out of group struggles over socially valued resources. They are systems of power relationships that are historically specific, socially constructed hierarchies of domination—not merely differences in cultural preferences, lifestyle choices, or rankings on a continuum of material resources. These social systems are embedded and have meaning in the micro level of individuals' everyday lives as well as in the macro levels of community and social institutions. The broad macro-level forces that shape events are remote and abstract and difficult to see. Race, class, gender, and sexuality simultaneously operate in every social situation and are concurrently experienced by individuals in their everyday lives.

To understand and effectively eliminate disparities requires a research methodology that recognizes the plurality, situational character, and interactive nature of factors (e.g., race, class, gender) influencing health status (Shavers-Hornaday et al. 1997). The health status of people who are poor and/or minorities should be understood in relation to their race, class, gender, and other dimensions of social difference. The U.S. has difficulty viewing difference without hierarchy (Zambrana 1987). It is easier and less controversial to talk about culture and language than to talk about literacy, poverty, and inequity. Many shy away from the language that defines the illness of racism that is linked to both access and quality of care for people of color and those living in poverty (Lillie-Blanton et al. 2000; Zambrana and Logie 2000; Jones 2000).

In the United States, most health promotion efforts focus on a narrow range of behaviors: tobacco use, alcohol/drug abuse, unhealthy diet, sedentary lifestyle, and risky sexual practices. Broader views of health promotion such as those supported by the World Health Organization are overshadowed by what individuals can do to protect their own health (Ruzek 1997). Current thinking about health in the U.S. begins with the assumption that women and racial/ethnic minorities and persons living in poverty have what the World Health Organization describes as the prerequisites for health (Ruzek, Oleson, and Clarke 1997; World Health Organization 1994). The prerequisites, outlined by Sheryl Ruzek (Ruzek 1995) in her address at the Society for Behavioral Medicine, include: freedom from the fear of war [or violence]; equal opportunity for all; satisfaction of basic needs for food, education, water, and sanitation; decent housing; secure work; a useful role in society; political will; and public support. Ruzek (Ruzek 1995) contends that these familiar components are building blocks of health that remain submerged in dominant biomedical and psychosocial models of health. In her Interdependent Model of Optimal Community Health, Ruzek (Ruzek 1995) emphasizes that health is not embedded in individual bodies but rather in social relationships that cultivate a shared sense of community.

The perspectives presented by Weber and Ruzek address the nature and importance of social context in health research. According to Smedley and Syme (Smedley and Syme 2000), social context is comprised of socioeconomic conditions and factors in one's physical, social, and cultural environment that influence access to health information, social support, social networks, social norms, and cultural beliefs and attitudes regarding health (Smedley and Syme 2000). It is important to study the social context in which behaviors occur. Research is needed to identify ways in which social context influences health behavior, environmental exposures, psychosocial responses, and health outcomes and mediates the influence of interventions.

The social context can influence health and health risk both directly or indirectly. Interventions must not only be adapted to differences in social context; they must also directly influence the social context. One aspect of social context that has increasingly gained attention in health behavior research is social capital. Social capital is an attribute of social structures (e.g., organizations, communities, neighborhoods, extended families) rather than individuals. It is a community-level measure of the quality of social relationships that facilitate the achievement of the collective goals of individuals within a community (Smedley and Syme 2000; Coleman

1990; Putnam 1993; Kawachi, Kennedy, and Glass 1999). Poverty has multiple effects not only on the individual, but also on his/her community. People in poverty-stricken communities do not have the resources to help one another; as a result, there is little trust or collaboration in those communities. Social capital provides a framework for evaluating the cohesiveness of communities and the resources available in those communities (Baum 1999; Kawachi 1999) to resolve problems.

Rather than focusing on a single or limited number of health determinants, interventions on social and behavioral factors should link multiple levels of influence. This leads to a significant change in the way that we conceptualize health behavior research and develop health promotion interventions. Rather than focusing on intrapersonal and interpersonal interventions, the theories and methods most commonly used, future research with diverse populations should utilize ecological approaches to address health disparities. Intervention strategies must attend to aspects of the social context that may hinder or promote efforts at behavioral change and risk reduction. Accessibility, physical structure, social structures and policies, and media and cultural messages of products and behaviors vary for different groups of people (Cohen, Scribner, and Farley 2000). As an example of the targeting of racial/ethnic groups by industries that may contribute to health disparities, Alaniz (Alaniz 1998) found high concentrations of alcohol outlets and advertisements in low-income African-American and Latino neighborhoods. Modifying social capital of communities in these neighborhoods offers promise to enhance social contexts.

Ecological Models of Health

Although individual level interventions have been the most commonly used methods in health promotion research and practice, it is not accurate to argue that health promotion is practiced only at the individual behavioral level (Perry et al. 2000). Theories and models of health behavior that recognize the multiple levels of influence—ecological models—have been developed. The beginning of the ecological movement can be traced to the 1980s. Borrowing from a broad range of disciplines, from sociology to medical geography (Green, Richard, and Potvin 1996), these ecological frameworks involve interventions at the intrapersonal, interpersonal, institutional or organizational, community, and public policy levels. By including the social context, these models provide a framework to intervene and positively affect health behaviors beyond the individual level and reach larger groups of people with sustainable approaches (Cohen, Scribner, and Farley 2000). McKinley (McKinley 1995) has proposed that effective population-based behavior change requires simultaneous intervention efforts across the all levels presented in the ecological model. In their review of population-based health promotion Orleans and colleagues (Orleans et al. 1999) conclude that although examples of successful interventions at each level exist, there are few that address the multiple levels simultaneously.

One of the most widely used community-level models is that developed by McLeroy and colleagues (McLeroy et al. 1988). In this model, health promotion interventions target multiple levels of influence and the target population actively participates in the identification of problems in the community and collaborates to address issues. With the support of the community, changes in the environmental influences on health behavior lead to changes in the health behaviors of the individuals in the community.

A model for evaluating the needs of a segment of the population and for developing appropriate interventions is PRECEDE-PROCEED. This planning model addresses behavior change at multiple levels. The PRECEDE-PROCEED model by Green (1984) has received extensive application in health programs and focuses on factors that shape behavioral actions. In the first step of this model, the target population identifies the issues that need to be addressed. In addition to evaluating the influences of behavior and of the environment on behavior, PRECEDE-PROCEED also examines interpersonal, social, and organizational factors and policies during the planning stage.

At each stage of PRECEDE-PROCEED, predisposing, reinforcing, and enabling factors shape behavioral actions. Predisposing factors provide the motivation behind a behavior; at the individual level, they include knowledge, attitude, cultural beliefs, and readiness for change. Reinforcing factors come to play after a behavior has begun and provide continuing rewards or incentives; they contribute to repetition or persistence of behaviors. At the interpersonal level, social support, praise, and symptom relief might all be reinforcing factors. Enabling factors make it possible for motivation to be realized, that is, they "enable" persons to act on their predisposition; at the organizational and policy levels, they include available resources, supportive policies, and services (Green 1984).

All of the ecological models of health behavior converge on one defining point—they are broader and more inclusive than previous theories. Their expansiveness is also the reason for their underutilization. The ecological model of McLeroy and colleagues (McLeroy et al. 1988) and the PRECEDE-PROCEED model involve assessing and addressing needs across the social strata (Green 1984). The development, implementation, and evaluation of interventions are time-consuming and require a considerable amount of resources (Stokols 1996; Green, Richard, and Potvin 1996). In order to make ecological models practical, guidelines have been developed by Stokols (Stokols 1996) that provide concise explanations of the multiple levels in the model. By using the four factors of availability, physical structures, social structures, and cultural and media messages addressed in Cohen and colleagues' (Cohen, Scribner, and Farley 2000) structural model, interventions based on ecological frameworks can be developed in a manageable format that will change the external factors and lead to positive behavioral changes in a specific subset of the population.

Conclusion

Individual-level behavior change approaches should not be abandoned in the search for an exclusive focus on societal solutions to health problems, but rather should become integrated within population-level approaches (Emmons 2000; Ruzek 1997). We cannot ignore the phenomenon of agency—the capacity of individuals to act on their own behalf in ways that meet their own needs. However, what individuals can do within their own personal spheres of influence to improve their own health and that of their community warrants more attention. Self-mastery, gaining control over personal health, may be the necessary first step to empowering individuals to bring about wider social change. If we are to adequately address health disparities, individual and societal responsibilities for health should be viewed as complementary. Interventions are needed that integrate strategies for dealing with social factors with those developed for individual-level change. We must work with communities to integrate social context into interventions that are meaningful and focus on increasing social capital. Behavior is inextricably linked to a larger social, political, and economic environment. If we continue to address public health problems without attending to the context in which they exist, we will not achieve our goal of eliminating health disparities.

References

Ajzen I, Fishbein M. *Understanding attitudes and Predicting Social Behaviors*. Englewood Cliffs, N.J.: Prentice-Hall; 1980.

Alaniz ML. Alcohol availability and targeted advertising in racial/ethnic minority communities. *Alcohol Health & Research World*. 1998;22:286-290.

Auslander W, Haire-Joshu D, Houston C, Williams, JH, Krebill H. The short-term impact of a health promotion program for low-income African American women. *Res Soc Work Pract*. 2000;10:78-97.

Bandura A. Perceived self-efficacy in the exercise of personal agency. *Psychologist: Bull Br Psychological Soc*. 1989;10:411-424.

Bandura A. Social cognitive theory of self regulation. *Organizational Behavior and Human Decision Processes*. 1991;50:248-285.

Bandura A. *Social Foundations of Thought and Action: A Social Cognitive Theory*. Englewood Cliffs, N.J.: Prentice Hall; 1986.

Baum F. Social Capital: Is it good for your health? Issues for a public health agenda. *J Epidemiol Community Health*. 1999;53:195-196.

Becker MH. The health belief model and personal health behavior. *Health Education Monographs*. 1974;2:324-508.

Cohen DA, Scribner RA, Farley TA. A structural model of health behavior: A pragmatic approach to explain and influence health behaviors at the population level. *Prev Med*. 2000;30:146-154.

Coleman JS. *The Foundations of Social Theory*. Cambridge, Mass.: Harvard University Press; 1990.

Council of Scientific Affairs. Hispanic health in the United States. *JAMA*. 1991;262:248-257.

Elder JP, Apodaca JX, Parra-Medina D, Zuniga de Nuncio ML. Strategies for health education: Theoretical models. In: Loue S, ed. *Handbook of Immigrant Health*. New York: Plenum Press; 1998:567-585.

Emmons KM. Behavioral and social science contributions to the health of adults in the United States. In: Smedley BD, Syme SL, eds. *Promoting Health: Intervention Strategies from Social and Behavioral Research*. Washington, D.C.: National Academy Press; 2000:254-321.

Fishbein M, Ajzen I. *Belief, Attitude, Intention and Behavior: An Introduction to Theory and Research*. Reading, Mass.: Addison-Wesley; 1975.

Fishbein M. A theory of Reasoned Action: Some applications and implications. In: Howe H, Page M, eds. *Nebraska Symposium on Motivation, 1979*. Lincoln: University of Nebraska Press; 1980:65–116.

Green LW. Modifying and developing health behavior. *Annu Rev Public Health*. 1984;5:215-236.

Green LW, Richard L, Potvin L. Ecological foundations of health promotion. *Am J Health Promotion*. 1996;10:270-281.

House JS, Williams DR. Understanding and reducing socioeconomic and racial/ethnic disparities in health. In: Smedley BD, Syme SL, eds. *Promoting Health: Intervention Strategies from Social and Behavioral Research*. Washington, D.C.: National Academy Press; 2000:81-124.

Janz NK, Becker MH. The health belief model: A decade later. *Health Education Q*. 1984;11:1-47.

Jones CP. Levels of racism: A theoretic framework and a gardener's tale. *Am J Public Health.* 2000;90:1212–1215.

Kawachi I. Social capital and community effects on population and individual health. *Ann N Y Acad Sci.* 1999;896:120–130.

Kawachi I, Kennedy BP, Glass R. Social capital and self-rated health: A contextual analysis. *Am J Public Health.* 1999;87:1497–1498.

LaVeist TA. Beyond dummy variables and sample selection: What health services researchers ought to know about race as a variable. *Health Serv Res.* 1994;29:1–16.

Lillie-Blanton M, Brodie M, Rowland D, Altman D, McIntosh M. Race, ethnicity, and the health care system: public perceptions and experiences. *Med Care Res Rev.* 2000;57:218–236.

Loue S. *Gender, Ethnicity, and Health Research.* New York: Kluwer Academic/Plenum Publishers; 1999.

Masi R, Mensah L, McLeod KA. *Health Cultures: Policies, Professional Practice and Education, Volume 1.* London: Mosaic Press; 1995.

McKinley J. The new public health approach to improving physical activity and autonomy in older populations. In: Heikkinon E, ed. *Preparation for Aging.* New York: Plenum; 1995.

McLeroy K, Bibeau D, Stecker A, Glanz K. An ecological perspective on health promotion programs. *Health Education Quarterly.* 1988;15:351–377.

National Institutes of Health. *Strategic Plan to Reduce and Ultimately Eliminate Health Disparities: Strategic Plan 2002–2006;* Draft October 6, 2000.

Orleans CT, Gruman J, Ulmer, Emont SL, Hollendonner JK. Rating our progress in population health promotion: Report Card on six behaviors. *Am J Health Promotion.* 1999;14(2):75–82.

Perry CL, Williams CL, Komro KA, Veblen-Mortenson S, Forster J, Bernstein-Lachter R, Pratt LK, Dudovitz B, Munson KA, Farbakhash K, Finnegan J, McGovern P. Project Northland high school interventions: Community action to reduce adolescent alcohol use. *Health Educ Behav.* 2000:27(1):29–49.

Prochaska J, DiClemente C. Stages and processes of self-change in smoking: Toward an integrative model of change. *J Consult Clin Psychol.* 1983;51:390–395.

Putnam RD. The prosperous community, Social capital and economic growth. *American Prospect.* 1993; Spring:35–42.

Rivara F P, Finberg L. Use of the terms Race and Ethnicity. *Arch Pediatr Adolesc Med.* 2001;155:119.

Rosenstock I. Historical origins of the health belief model. *Health Education Monographs.* 1974;2:328–335.

Rosenstock I. Why people use health services. *Millbank Memorial Fund Q.* 1966;44:94–124.

Ruzek, SB. Caring, curing and concern: Key concepts for an integrated model of women's health. In: *Beyond Diseases: Forging an Integrated Model of Women's Health.* March 25, 1995. Symposium conducted at the Annual Meeting of the Society of Behavioral Medicine, San Diego.

Ruzek SB. Women, personal health behavior, and health promotion. In: Ruzek SB, Oleson VL, Clarke AC, eds. *Women's Health: Complexities and Differences.* Columbus: Ohio State University Press; 1997:118–153.

Ruzek SB, Oleson VL, Clarke AC. Social, Biomedical, and Feminist Models of Women's Health. In: Ruzek SB, Oleson VL, Clarke AC, eds. *Women's Health: Complexities and Differences.* Columbus: Ohio State University Press; 1997:11–28.

Senior PA, Bhopal R. Ethnicity as a variable in epidemiological research. *British Med J.* 1994; 309:327–330.

Shavers-Hornaday VL, Lynch CF, Burmeister LF, Torner JC. Why are African Americans underrepresented in medical research studies? Impediments to participation. *Ethn Health.* 1997;2:31–45.

Smedley BD, Syme SL. Promoting health: Intervention strategies from social and behavioral research. In: Smedley BD, Syme SL, eds. *Promoting Health: Intervention Strategies from Social and Behavioral Research.* Washington, D.C.: National Academy Press; 2000:1–36.

Stokols D. Translating Social Ecological Theory into guidelines for community health promotion. *Am J Health Promotion.* 1996;10:282–298.

United States Department of Health and Human Services. *Healthy People 2010: Understanding and Improving Health.* 2nd ed. Washington, D.C.: U.S. Government Printing Office; Nov. 2000.

Wallack L. The role of mass media in creating social capital: A new direction for public health. In: Smedley BD, Syme SL, eds. *Promoting Health: Intervention Strategies from Social and Behavioral Research*. Washington, D.C.: National Academy Press; 2000:337–365.

Weber L. *Understanding Race, Class, Gender, and Sexuality: A Conceptual Framework*. Boston: McGraw-Hill; 2001.

Weber L, Hancock T, Higginbotham E. Women, power, and mental health. In: Ruzek SB, Oleson VL, Clarke AC, eds. *Women's Health: Complexities and Differences*. Columbus: Ohio State University Press; 1997:380–396.

Williams DR. Race and health: Basic questions, emerging directions. *Ann Epidemiol*. 1997;7:322–333.

Williams DR, Collins C. U.S. socioeconomic and racial differences in health: Patterns and explanations. *Annu Rev Sociol*. 1995;21:349–386.

World Health Organization. *Women's Health Counts: Vienna Statement on Investing in Women's Health in the Countries of Central and Eastern Europe*. Copenhagen: WHO Regional Office for Europe; 1994.

Zambrana RE. A research agenda on issues affecting poor and minority women: A model for understanding their health needs. *Women Health*. 1987;Winter:137–160.

Zambrana RE, Logie LA. Latino child health: Need for inclusion in the U.S. national discourse. *Am J Public Health*. 2000;90:1827–1834.

Chapter 7

GENETIC RESEARCH *with* MINORITY POPULATIONS

Morris W. Foster, PhD,
and Richard R. Sharp, PhD

Before the technology to analyze DNA existed, genetic researchers had a long history of recruiting participants from small, socially defined populations, many of which could be considered minority communities. Efforts to identify Mendelian disorders, for example, frequently examined populations that had experienced geographic isolation or population bottlenecks, or had historic patterns of in-marriage (http://www3.ncbi.nlm.nih.gov/Omim/). These populations, such as the Amish or Ashkenazi Jews (Egelund and Hostetter 1983; Bundey, Harrison, and Marsden 1975), were socially identifiable to outsiders; many had historical experiences of discrimination or stigmatization, often based on perceptions of biological differences that were reified as racial or ethnic categories. Nonetheless, geneticists were able to establish long-term relationships with discrete local communities within these minority populations, some of which led to the identification and characterization of several genetic disorders.

Not all genetic research with socially defined populations has been as successful. A prominent example was the identification of sickle cell trait among African-Americans. Although not limited to African-Americans, the association of the recessive genetic variant for sickle cell disease with a socially defined racial category resulted in discriminatory policies and stigmatizing attitudes (Duster 1990). The experience of sickle cell research was evidence of the potential for genetic findings to be used to reinforce the mistaken idea that social identities such as race and ethnicity have an underlying biological basis.

In part, the different historical experiences of genetic research among socially identifiable populations are a function of scale and approach. Amish and Ashkenazi populations are much smaller than the African-American population. Genetic studies among the former constitute a type of pedigree study, taking advantage of the relative reproductive isolation of select families comprising the population. It is this relative isolation that enabled researchers to use the distinctive social identities of these populations to follow rare genetic variants from one generation to another. Genetic studies among larger, more heterogeneous populations, however, used allelic frequency to identify common, but by no means ubiquitous, genetic features. Pedigree studies of rare disorders may be less likely to stigmatize everyone who shares the same social identity as members of the affected family, while population studies of common disorders are more likely to have implications for all who share that social label. Many pedigree studies, though, do name the populations in which affected families are situated, creating the potential for associating all members of a population with diseases for which most are not at risk. Similarly, population genetic studies sometimes initially identify a population as at higher risk for a disease before later determining that the higher risk is confined to a previously unidentified pedigree within the larger population (Arnet et al. 1996; Tan et al. 1998).

Genetic research, of course, does not exist in a political or historical vacuum. The broader social experiences of a racial or ethnic population with the dominant society also shape the response of the minority population to opportunities to participate in research. Not surprisingly, members of communities that are more politically aware of the effects of European colonization and domination are the least likely to volunteer for genetic studies or clinical trials; African-Americans and Native Americans, for example, have expressed reservations about genetic research and the uses to which findings about their DNA might be put (Mogilner et al. 1998; Dukepoo 1998). This legacy of mistrust stems from other African-American and Native American experiences of the use of biological claims to treat them as socially distinct categories of people.

Studying a Shared Genetic Heritage, Searching for Difference

In its initial formulation, the Human Genome Project (HGP), a multinational effort to sequence all genetic information contained on human chromosomes, promised to put an end to perceptions of biological differences among human populations (Gilbert 1992). The HGP would do so in two ways: first, by demonstrating that all humans share a common DNA sequence (often referred to as "The Book of Life" by HGP proponents), and second, by individualizing medical practice so that racial and ethnic disparities based on assumptions of biological difference no longer exist (the cost of and access to individualized medical care would, of course, continue to be a social problem). In the mid-1990s, when large-scale DNA sequencing was under way, HGP leaders were fond of noting that 99.9% of human genes are shared in common by every individual, regardless of race or ethnicity (Guyer and Collins 1995). Over the same period, rapidly improving DNA-based technologies moved closer toward the capability of testing a single sample for multiple genetic variants—the basis for individualized diagnosis and therapy.

Population geneticists and physical anthropologists, concerned that human genetic diversity was being ignored, criticized the HGP's initial emphasis on the commonality of genetic features (Cavalli-Sforza et al. 1991). Identifying this genetic diversity, which they believed was distributed unevenly among different socially defined populations, was of special interest to population geneticists in light of what they believed to be increasing admixture between historically isolated populations. In response, a group of concerned scientists proposed what came to be known as the Human Genome Diversity Project (HGDP) (Human Genome Diversity Committee 1994). A central goal of the HGDP was to use DNA collected from socially defined populations around the world to decipher human population histories and patterns of migration. Although the HGDP never developed into an ongoing, centrally coordinated, government-funded effort, it did attract pilot funding and support from the international Human Genome Organization (HUGO), the MacArthur Foundation, and the National Science Foundation (NSF). While individual HGDP supporters continued to assemble and maintain population-specific collections of genetic materials, a common HGDP repository was never established.

In spite of the HGDP's failure as a "Big Science" project, the concept of a centralized "genetic diversity project" galvanized concerns about population-specific genetic research (Rothman 1998). Those concerns ranged from worries about reifying social identities as biological categories, to questions of subject exploitation and commercial interests, to difficulties arising from the potential for genetic studies to undermine a population's traditional views of its origin and history. In addition to these concerns about the HGDP, critics of the project alleged that it had conflated population history research (which primarily benefits researchers) with biomedical research (which could benefit populations being studied) (Foster and Freeman 1998). These ambiguities made it difficult to evaluate both the scientific value of the HGDP as well as its potential risks and benefits (Committee on Human Genome Diversity 1997). In response, the HGDP developed a model ethical protocol for collecting biological materials from discrete populations (North American Regional Committee of the Human Genome Diversity Project 1997). Nonetheless, while the model ethical protocol provided guidelines for evaluating some concerns, others, like the control of future uses of samples and the return of benefit to participating communities, remained largely unexamined.

Many indigenous communities and advocacy organizations perceived the HGDP as a colonialist enterprise (National Congress of American Indians 1998), often extending these criticisms to genetic and genomic research in general (Indigenous Peoples Coalition Against Biopiracy 1996). Proponents of the HGP and related biomedical projects carefully avoided association with the HGDP and were vocal in their criticism of inappropriate biological uses of social categories such as race and ethnicity. The focus of the HGP on health research and its emphasis on shared genetic features (as opposed to features specific to certain populations) were contrasted to the HGDP and the later project's interest in identifying genetic differences between populations.

However, by 1997, changes in genomic science and technology made sequence variation an increasingly important focus (Collins, Guyer, and Chakravarti 1997). Because all humans share approximately 99.9% of the same genes, disease genes for rare Mendelian disorders (such as sickle cell and cystic fibrosis) and highly predictive susceptibility genes for complex disorders (such as cancer and diabetes) must be located in the 0.1% that are not shared by everyone. Hence, if the HGP were to have a medical payoff once the entire genome was sequenced, a significant part of the post-genomic focus necessarily would be on inter-individual sequence variation (Collins 1999). This new emphasis would create a tension between the common humanity the HGP originally promised to reveal and the search for genetic differences contributing to illness and disease.

A central locus for the investigation of genetic difference is single nucleotide polymorphisms (SNPs). SNPs are variations in single DNA bases on the long chains of millions of DNA base pairs that comprise the chromosomes. Some SNPs appear to have no functional consequences, but others have functional implications that make people who possess them more susceptible to particular diseases than others. In the case of a complex disease such as diabetes, for instance, multiple SNPs appear to be required to predispose an individual to that disease (Pederson 1999). It also appears that more than one combination of different SNPs may lead to similar diabetic predispositions (Mathews and Berdanier 1998). Consequently, in studying a disease such as diabetes, it makes sense to analyze DNA from diabetics who are more likely to be biologically related to one another—because they are more likely to share the same combination of SNPs that lead to their particular variety of diabetes. Moreover, analyses of biologically related participants who have and do not have diabetes also greatly reduces the amount of genetic "noise" that often results from spurious genetic associations that have nothing to do with diabetes. Thus, studying biologically related participants continues to offer genetic researchers analytic advantages over the study of unrelated individuals. These advantages make it likely that pedigree studies and studies of small minority populations consisting of several extended families will continue to play an important role in DNA research.

Ethical and Scientific Aspects of the Use of Race and Ethnicity in Genetic Research

The analytic advantages of studying biologically related participants sometimes incur social costs. For example, when researchers use social categories to recruit participants they may inadvertently confuse the relationship between socially defined populations from which study participants are recruited and biological characteristics of those populations, assuming that the path between the two is more direct than it in fact is. With regard to analysis of siblings and family members (who are likely to share most genetic variants) and pedigree analysis, the biological basis for recruiting members of the same socially defined family is fairly well specified. Some degree of false paternity and fictive kinship may confound the relationship, but otherwise such studies raise few ethical challenges. Additional protection for participants and their families can be obtained by not releasing family names, thereby limiting potential harms that may result from mapping genetic predispositions for disease onto identifiable social units such as families.

The use of social categories as a proxy for biological relatedness becomes somewhat more opaque when extra-familial social identities such as race and ethnicity are used as research variables. While the degree of relatedness will be less than in the case of pedigrees and siblings, the assumption is that members of such socially defined populations have some greater likelihood of genetic similarity because of a shared ancestral history. That biological relatedness may be reinforced by preferential in-marriage, population bottlenecks, and geographic isolation. Thus, it is not unusual for geneticists to speak of allelic frequencies, polymorphic variants, and even genetic disorders as being specific to particular ethnic or racial populations (McLeod et al. 1999; Weber 1999). As a consequence of this mode of thinking, participants in genetic studies often are recruited based on their social identities, either as a way of obtaining a large number of individuals who are likely to have a particular disease or genetic polymorphism, or as a way of reducing the background noise—or both. Moreover, population-based genetic studies almost always publish participants' social identities, exposing all persons who share those recognizable labels to harms resulting from the association of a social category with a biological trait (Foster and Sharp 2000).

Genetic variation undoubtedly accounts for some part of the uneven distribution of burdens for specific diseases both within and between socially defined populations (Shriver 1997). Similarly, some differences in response to therapeutic drugs and environmental toxins also may be accounted for by sequence variation within and between such populations (Hall et al. 1999). The challenge for genetic researchers is to determine how such social categories correspond to biological functions. Thus, two central questions suggest themselves: 1) How to interpret associations between genetic variants and the increased prevalence of a disease, therapeutic effect, or environmental response within the social categories in which we are accustomed to classifying people, and 2) How to investigate those differences in ways that are sensitive to cultural differences and minimize potential harms to socially defined populations. These problems are presently being debated by bioethicists, policy makers, and others involved in the protection of human subjects in research. They are perhaps best understood by surveying the primary issues that have been raised in that emerging literature.

Are Race and Ethnicity Scientific Categories?

Most social scientists and some health researchers have argued that race and ethnicity are, primarily, social categories that have no biological reality (Sheldon and Parker 1992; Anand 1999; Dyson 1998; Freeman 1998). The first chapter in this volume by Williams and Rubio provides an in-depth discussion of the meaning of race in research. Intermarriage, cultural preferences for claiming only a father's or a mother's identity, fictive kinship, instrumental and situational choices in asserting identity, and colonialist, racist, and nationalist ideologies that impose new identities on subjugated populations are but a few of the social mechanisms that make social identities poor proxies for biological relatedness. Nonetheless, many genetic studies continue to use race and ethnicity as inclusion criteria for participant recruitment. Most studies also use race and ethnicity as variables in analyzing or reporting genetic findings. With few exceptions, racial and ethnic identities of participants in those studies are based on uninvestigated self-representations, resulting in poorly defined analytic categories.

Uses of social identities in research can be more rigorous, however (Foster, Sharp, and Mulvihill 2001). Social identities can be investigated and detailed family histories taken, thus providing more accurate proxies for biological relatedness. Alternatively, self-representation of social identity may be a critical scientific variable in assessing the significance of race and ethnicity as social phenomena. Thus, even in cases where racial or ethnic categories are poor proxies for biological relatedness, such variables may serve an important role in scientific analyses, for example, as proxies for cultural practices, social advantage or disadvantage, experiences of racism, behavior, or diet.

Recruitment and Analysis

It may be helpful to separate the uses of race and ethnicity in recruiting study participants from their uses in analyzing genetic findings. Some genetic studies use social identity as a criterion for participant recruitment to take advantage of already reported higher epidemiological frequencies of a particular disease or polymorphism in a given population. In that sense, using social identity is a practical method for obtaining a convenient sample of appropriate participants, and self-representation of that identity may be sufficient to attract appropriate volunteers. In fact, participants in many genetic studies comprise convenience samples rather than samples that are representative of either local or national socially defined populations. Difficulties arise when researchers fail to appreciate this, and so go on to use these social identities to analyze their genetic data (Foster and Sharp 2002). Thus, findings are reported as "African-American" or "Mexican American" even though those categorizations are primarily social artifacts of how participants were recruited.

A scientifically appropriate standard for using race or ethnicity to analyze genetic data would require that researchers demonstrate that their participant sample is representative of the larger socially defined population in question. Only then would the findings be demographically and clinically applicable to broad ethnic and racial categories. This, however, raises the further question of the hierarchical nature of many social identities within a population. The findings for a local African-American population or a particular Native American tribe may not be applicable to other localities or tribes or to African-Americans in a particular state or region or Native Americans in the same language family or to all African-Americans or all Native Americans. As the specificity and scale of the socially defined population changes, so too may research findings, which is additional reason to examine the use of racial and ethnic categories as both recruitment and analytic variables.

Inclusion, Reification, and Significance

As a matter of public policy, Congress has mandated that federally funded health research should include members of minority populations so that those populations will share in the benefits of research findings. As a matter of research practice, however, such inclusion has the potential to perpetuate the assumption that racial and ethnic identities have a biological basis. This is because minority inclusion requirements often are interpreted to mandate that a study include minority participants in proportion to their representation in the local population(s) from which other participants are recruited. Often, this means that minority participants are included in numbers too small to reach statistical significance and in a manner that does not ensure that they are representative of local or national populations. When researchers interpret the policy mandate as license to analyze and report genetic findings using racial and ethnic identities, the result is the reification of social categories as biologically meaningful.

An alternative approach is to avoid using and reporting racial and ethnic categories unless there is a compelling scientific rationale for doing otherwise. This is the stance taken by the Polymorphism Discovery Resource (PDR), a collection of DNA samples assembled to represent the range of genetic diversity within the U.S. population (Collins, Brooks, and Chakravarti 1998). The racial and ethnic identities of PDR sample donors are not provided to users of the collection, and users are explicitly precluded from trying to identify those identities as a condition of use. Thus, the PDR allows researchers to investigate a wide range of biological diversity without filtering genetic variation through the lens of pre-existing social categories.

Public Health Benefits and Risks

Despite questions about the scientific significance of social identities for research studies, their significance for public health purposes remains compelling. The continuing social relevance of race and ethnicity makes such identities powerful means for communicating public health information. Thus, awareness of sickle cell trait among African-Americans and of Tay Sachs among Ashkenazi Jews has had, arguably, a beneficial effect in understanding, preventing, and treating those genetic disorders, even though the disorders are not restricted to those populations, nor is everyone in those populations equally at risk (Andrews et al. 1994). At the same time, public health uses of racial and ethnic identities also may be exclusionary and stigmatizing. Diagnoses of sickle cell and cystic fibrosis, for instance, often are missed or delayed when patients are not identified as being members of higher risk racial or ethnic populations (Shafer et al. 1996; Spencer et al. 1994). Being a member of what is publicly labeled as a higher-risk population also can lead to a shared stigmatization, as already noted in the case of sickle cell trait, even though one is neither a carrier nor an affected.

Community Review and Involvement

Genetic research can present unique challenges for the protection of human subjects, raising difficult issues of collective risks and benefits that cannot be addressed fully through individual informed consent and review by institution review boards. This has catalyzed the development of innovative efforts to involve communities in the design and review of genetic studies (Foster, Eisenbraun, and Carter 1997). Initial experiences in conducting community review in Native American tribes suggest that outsiders often cannot anticipate local perceptions of risks and benefits (Foster et al. 1999). Frequently, the more prominent local concerns about a genetic study focus on how its conduct and findings may disrupt relationships among community members rather than on how information about the community may be used by outsiders. While Native American tribes are sovereign entities and are politically organized to provide formal consent for conducting genetic studies among their members (or to decline such studies), other kinds of communities lack similar central public authorities. In those latter cases, different forms of community involvement can be undertaken to give community members a voice in how a study is designed and how individual participants and supporting communities are protected (Sharp and Foster 2000).

Community involvement is complicated by hierarchically nested identities that may require multiple levels of consultation, geographic dispersion of some socially defined populations into multiple communities, other populations that are comprised of geographically overlapping communities, persons who share a social identity but do not choose to be members of communities that are organized around that label, and the concomitant requirement to respect the autonomous choice of individuals to participate in a study or not (Juengst 1998). Among the issues commonly negotiated with communities in the context of genetic research are control of future uses of DNA samples, reporting study findings to supporting communities, incorporation of research questions that may be of interest to community members, provision of health benefits, funding community organizations and individuals to conduct parts of the study, and sharing any commercial royalties from study discoveries. Despite the many challenges involved, community involvement is, perhaps, the most promising mechanism for encouraging minority populations to participate in genetic research, and for empowering them in doing so (Sharp and Foster 2002a).

Conclusion

As these and other issues are identified, explored, and debated, scientific and ethical standards for the use of social identities in genetic research will continue to evolve (Sharp and Foster 2002b). Two recent examples of such changes are a requirement for community consultation before population-specific samples can be deposited in a national biological repository supported by the National Institutes of Health (http://locus.umdnj.edu/nigms/comm/submit/collpolicy.html) and a requirement for scientific justification before a population can be identified in articles published in a prominent genetics journal (Census, race, and science, Nat Genet 2000). In addition, the Ethical, Legal, and Social Implications (ELSI) program of the National Human Genome Research Institute (NHGRI), the principal U.S. organization supporting the HGP, has made the investigation of genetic variation research one of its top funding priorities (http://www.hngri.nih.gov/ELSI). Some population geneticists are beginning to appreciate that genomic diversity does not correspond directly to social, cultural, or linguistic divergence (Harding 2000).

Still, genetics research clearly presents more risks for minority populations than for the dominant population. Racism and ethnic nationalism historically have been justified by appeals to biological difference. Race and ethnicity, although demonstrably social categories, continue to be uncritically assumed to imply biological relatedness by many geneticists, who frequently use self-reported social identities as convenient means to recruit study participants and analyze data. Epidemiologists' habit of representing disease risk through social identities, though offering some compelling public health benefits, further perpetuates the geneticization of racial and ethnic categories (Oppenheimer 2001).

At the same time, minority populations have much to gain from the clinical applications that one day will flow from post-genomic research. For example, pharmacogenetics, the study of genetic influences on drug response, will likely allow drugs to be tailored to the genotypes of individual patients, increasing therapeutic efficacy and minimizing adverse response (Wolf, Smith, and Smith 2000). Similarly, toxicogenetics, the study of genetic influences on the metabolism of environmental toxins, will give public health officials a much better understanding of who is most vulnerable to various occupational and environmental agents, perhaps leading to the development of more effective disease prevention programs (Nuwaysir et al. 1999). While many patterns of pharmaceutical and environmental response will not be racially or ethnically specific, the failure to include significant numbers of minority participants in clinical research leading to their development may result in some part of the range of genetic variation in drug response or toxic exposure not being included in product and testing development. Similarly, clinicians may be uncertain about the applicability of DNA-based diagnostics and therapeutics for populations that have not been involved in research development.

Finally, even if the scientific limitations and ethical risks of using social identities in genetic research are resolved, those solutions will not end the use of race and ethnicity in other aspects of our daily lives. As a result, social identity will continue to be a significant contributor to environmental factors affecting health (such as behavior, diet, and access to healthcare services). Thus, to the extent that racial and ethnic identities serve as salient proxies for non-genetic influences on illness and disease, the investigation of those social categories will continue to constitute an important complement to genetic research.

Acknowledgements

This publication was made possible by grant number ES11174 from the National Institute of Environmental Health Sciences (NIEHS) and the National Human Genome Research Institute (NHGRI). Its contents are solely the responsibility of the authors and do not necessarily represent the official views of the NIEHS, the NHGRI, or the National Institutes of Health.

References

Anand SS. Using ethnicity as a classification variable in health research: perpetuating the myth of biological determinism, serving socio-political agendas, or making valuable contributions to medical sciences? *Ethnicity Health*. 1999;4:241-244.

Andrews LB, Fullarton JE, Holtzman NA, Motulsky AG, eds. *Assessing genetic risks: implications for health and social policy*. Washington, D.C.: National Academies Press; 1994.

Arnett FC, Howard RF, Tan F, Moulds JM, Bias WB, Durban E, et al. Increased prevalence of systemic sclerosis in a Native American tribe in Oklahoma: association with an Amerindian haplotype. *Arthritis Rheum* 1996;39:1362-1370.

Bundey S, Harrison MJ, Marsden CD. A genetic study of torsion dystonia. *J Med Genet* 1975;12:12-19.

Cavalli-Sforza LL, Wilson AC, Cantor CR, Cook-Deegan RM, King M-C. Call for a worldwide survey of human genetic diversity: a vanishing opportunity for the Human Genome Project. *Genomics* 1991;11:490-91.

Census, race, and science [editorial]. *Nat Genet* 2000;24:97-98.

Collins FS. Shattuck lecture: medical and societal consequences of the Human Genetics Project. *N Engl J Med* 1999;341:28-36.

Collins FS, Brooks LD, Chakravarti A. A DNA polymorphism discovery resource for research on human genetic variation. *Genome Res* 1998;8:1229-1231.

Collins FS, Guyer MS, Chakravarti A. Variations on a theme: cataloging human DNA sequence variation. *Science* 1997;278:1580-1581.

Committee on Human Genome Diversity, National Research Council. *Evaluating human genetic diversity.* Washington, D.C.: National Academy of Science; 1997.

Dukepoo FC. Commentary on "Scientific limitations and ethical ramifications of non-representative Human Genome Project: African American Responses": an American Indian perspective. *Sci Eng Ethics* 1998;4:171-80.

Duster T. *Backdoor to eugenics.* New York: Rutledge; 1990.

Dyson SM. "Race," ethnicity and haemoglobin disorders. *Soc Sci Med* 1998;47:121-131.

Egelund JA, Hostetter AM. Amish study I: affective disorders among the Amish, 1976-1980. *Am J Psychiatry* 1983;140:57-61.

Foster MW, Eisenbraun AJ, Carter TH. Communal discourse as a supplement to informed consent in Genetic Research. *Nat Genet* 1997;17:277-279.

Foster MW, Freeman WL. Naming names in human genetic variation research. *Genome Res* 1998;8:755-757.

Foster MW, Sharp RR. Genetic research and culturally specific risks: one size does not fit all. *Trends Genet* 2000;16:93-95.

Foster MW, Sharp RR. Race, ethnicity, and genomics: social classifications as proxies for biological heterogeneity. *Genome Res* 2002;12:844-850.

Foster MW, Sharp RR, Mulvihill JJ. Pharmacogenetics, race, and ethnicity: social identities and individualized medical care. *Ther Drug Monitoring* 2001;23:232-238.

Foster MW, Sharp RR, Freeman WL, Chino M, Bernsten D, Carter TH. The role of community review in evaluating the risks of human genetic variation research. *Am J Hum Genet* 1999;64:1719-1727.

Freeman HP. The meaning of race in science—considerations for cancer research: concerns of special populations in the National Cancer Program. *Cancer* 1998;82:219-225.

Gilbert W. A vision of the grail. In: Kevles DJ, Hood L, eds. *The code of codes: scientific and social issues in the human genome project.* Cambridge, Mass.: Harvard; 1992.

Guyer MS, Collins FS. How is the Human Genome Project doing, and what have we learned so far? *Proc Natl Acad Sci U S A.* 1995;92:10841-10848.

Hall D, Ybazeta G, Destro-Bisol G, Petzl-Erler ML, Di Rienzo A. Variability at the uridine diphosphate glucuronosyltransferase 1A1 promoter in human populations and primates. *Pharmacogenetics* 1999;9:591-599.

Harding RM. Diversity, not divergence. *Trends Genet* 2000;16:381.

http://locus.umdnj.edu/nigms/comm/submit/collpolicy.html.

http://www.nhgri.nih.gov/ELSI/.

http://www3.ncbi.nlm.nih.gov/Omim/.

Human Genome Diversity Committee of the Human Genome Organisation. *The Human Genome Diversity Project, summary document.* London: Human Genome Organization; 1994.

Indigenous Peoples Coalition Against Biopiracy. Key points for a resolution condemning the Human Genome Diversity Project. Nixon, Nev.: Indigenous Peoples Coalition Against Biopiracy; 1996.

Juengst E. Groups as gatekeepers to genomic research: conceptually confusing, morally hazardous, and practically useless. *Kennedy Inst Ethics J* 1998;8:183-200.

Mathews CE, Berdanier CD. Noninsulin-dependent diabetes mellitus as a mitochondrial genomic disease. *Proc Soc Exp Biol Med* 1998;219:97-108.

McLeod HL, Pritchard SC, Githang'a J, Indalo A, Ameyaw MM, et al. Ethnic differences in thiopurine methyltansferase pharmacogenetics: evidence for allele specificity in Caucasian and Kenyan individuals. *Pharmacogenetics* 1999;9:773-776.

Mogilner A, Otten M, Cunningham JD, Brower ST. Awareness and attitudes concerning BRCA gene testing. *Ann Surg Oncol* 1998;5:607-12.

National Congress of American Indians. Resolution condemning the Human Genome Diversity Project (Res. No. NV-93-118). 1998.

North American Regional Committee of the Human Genome Diversity Project. Proposed model ethical protocol for collecting DNA samples. *Houston Law Review* 1997;33:1431-73.

Nuwaysir EF, Bittner M, Trent J, Barrett JC, Afshari CA. Microarrays and toxicology: the advent of toxicogenomics. *Mol Carcinog* 1999;24:153-159.

Oppenheimer GM. Paradigm lost: race, ethnicity, and the search for a new population taxonomy. *Am J Public Health* 2001;91:1049-1055.

Pedersen O. Genetics of insulin resistance. *Exp Clin Endocrinol Diabetes* 1999;107:113-118.

Rothman BK. *Genetic maps and the human imagination: the limits of science in understanding who we are.* New York: Norton; 1998.

Shafer FE, Lorey F, Cunningham GC, Klumpp C, Vichinsky E, Lubin B. Newborn screening for sickle cell disease: 4 years of experience from California's newborn screening program. *J Pediatr Hematol Oncol* 1996;18:36-41.

Sharp RR, Foster MW. An analysis of research guidelines on the collection and use of human biological materials from American Indian and Alaskan Native communities. *Jurimetrics* 2002a; 42:165-186.

Sharp RR, Foster MW. Community involvement in the ethical review of genetic research: lessons from American Indian and Alaska Native populations. *Environ Health Perspect.* 2002b;110(suppl 2):145-148.

Sharp RR, Foster MW. Involving study populations in the review of genetic research. *J Law Med Ethics* 2000;28:41-51.

Sheldon TA, Parker H. Race and ethnicity in health research. *J Public Health Med* 1992;14:104-110.

Shriver, MD. Ethnic variation as a key to the biology of human disease. *Ann Intern Med* 1997;127:401-403.

Spencer DA, Venkatataman M, Higgins S, Stevenson K, Weller PW. Cystic fibrosis in children from ethnic minorities in the West Midlands. *Respir Med* 1994;88:671-675.

Tan FK, Stivers DN, Foster MW, Chakraborty R, Howard RF, Milewicz DM, et al. Association of microsatellite markers near the fibrillin 1 gene on human chromosome 15q with scleroderma in a Native American population. *Arthritis Rheum* 1998;41:1729-37.

Weber WW. Populations and genetic polymorphisms. *Mol Diagn* 1999;4:299-307.

Wolf CR, Smith G, Smith RL. Pharmacogenetics. *BMJ* 2000;320:987-990.

Chapter 8

TRANSFORMING SCIENTIFIC INTERVENTION RESEARCH STRATEGIES *to Strengthen Community Capacity*

Collins O. Airhihenbuwa, PhD, MPH,
Leonard Jack, Jr., PhD, MS,
and J. DeWitt Webster, MPH, CHES

Introduction

The persistent gap in health status between White Americans and racial/ethnic minorities, particularly African-Americans, has intensified the interest in seeking policy and research strategies to close this gap. Efforts to address the persistent health disparities among African-Americans have resulted in a re-examination of current approaches to resolve health problems in this population. This re-examination hopefully will lead to a better understanding of the community contexts in which people of color live and work. Because the community context influences the capacity of African-Americans to participate in health intervention studies (Jack et al. 1999), defining community capacity will help establish a framework that can guide future outreach efforts and can increase the likelihood of participation by African-Americans in such studies.

A community is defined as the shared values, beliefs, and power relationships in a given entity that may have been mapped historically (Asante 1987; Airhihenbuwa 1995; Charatz-Litt 1991), politically (Freire 1973; Giroux 1992; Bernstein et al. 1994), professionally (Lupton 1994; Nickens 1985); culturally (Airhihenbuwa 1995; Airhihenbuwa 1994; Braithwaite and Lythcott 1989; Hahn 1995), and/or collectively through a coalition (Butterfoss, Goodman, and Wansersman 1993; Butterfoss,

Note: This chapter is based on a paper delivered by the first author at the American Public Health Association (APHA) annual meeting in Chicago, Illinois, November 9, 1999. A modified version of this paper was subsequently delivered at the 2000 mid-year scientific conference sponsored by the Association of State and Territorial Directors of Health Promotion and Public Health Education (ASTDHPPHE), the Society for Public Health Education (SOPHE), and Centers for Disease Control and Prevention (CDC).

Goodman, and Wansersman 1996). Capacity has emerged as a coupling designation in an attempt to debunk the traditional representation of community as a problem entity with deficits and minimal assets. Capacity engenders assets that allow the community to respond adequately to health issues and problems that may be social or political (Airhihenbuwa 1995; Braithwaite and Taylor 1992; Airhihenbuwa 1999; Green and Kreuter 1999). Thus, defining community capacity involves the assessment and evaluation of community (Goodman et al. 1998) as an entity whose resources include evident capabilities that should be the foundation for health interventions.

Determining community capacity among people of color would require identifying the community members' shared historical, political, and cultural values and beliefs. Such comprehensive evaluation encourages the assessment of both the assets and the liabilities of the community's capacity before initiating major components of the health intervention study. In this chapter, we will address the African-American community's capacity to participate in public health research and interventions. We will begin by exploring the background and challenges of involving African-American participants in public health research and interventions (including clinical trials), and we will examine methodological issues and their relevance to communities of color. We will conclude with recommendations for training public health professionals based on current research and interventions at the national and international levels.

Medical Victimization and Challenges to Participation in Health Intervention Studies

Public health, behavioral, and biomedical researchers are challenged to ensure adequate racial/ethnic minority representation in their study populations (Burrus, Liburd, and Burroughs 1998). Having proportionate numbers of minority participants ensures that data collection and study results adequately reflect the character of the diverse U.S. population. Study results that reflect ethnic representation are not only more generalizable, but also promote greater community acceptance, which are both necessary foundations for building effective culturally sensitive, age-appropriate health interventions. The National Institute of Health's (NIH) requirement for researchers to include minority representatives in their study populations, coupled with the persistent health disparities between racial/ethnic minorities and the White population, has intensified the search for strategies for recruiting and retaining ethnic minority populations in these studies; with the targeted minority population, older men and women, and populations with chronic illnesses and lower income are typically underrepresented (Patrick, Pruchno, and Rose 1998; Chadiha et al. 1994).

An underlying value of voluntary participation in medical research is the belief that the studies will result in new knowledge and/or products that will benefit the health of the participant, her/his family, and the greater community at large. Indeed, there is a high value placed on ultimate benefits to the community even if the participant does not benefit immediately. Unfortunately, past medical research practices in the United States have demonstrated that this assumption does not always hold true. In *Give Me My Father's Body: The Life of Minik, the New York Eskimo*, Ken Harper (2000) details the experience of six Polar Eskimos taken from their home in northwestern Greenland by Robert Peary, the North Pole explorer, to be studied. This experiment in anthropology brought three men, one woman, and two children from Smith Sound, Greenland, to New York in 1897 for the purpose of science and research. Their trip was preceded by the deaths of several Eskimos from Labrador, who were transported to the World's Colombian Exposition in Chicago in 1893; the bodies of these "exhibits" for science and the public voyeur became permanent museum collections after their deaths. Although this medical atrocity was before the Nuremberg code, the medical victimization of people of color and the institutionalized (Braslow 1996) is a part of current history in the U.S. In the book entitled *Acres of Skin*, Hornblum (Hornblum 1998) detailed "how American prisoners were exploited in the name of medical science just as senile hospital patients, retarded orphans, and other institutionalized populations were exploited in postwar America." The skins of inmates in Holmsburg prison in Philadelphia became the specimen on which the field of dermatology was to be advanced, irrespective of the inmates' consent or the physical and psychological devastation the experiment caused them. It would appear as though the Nuremberg code, crafted to protect research on human subjects, does not apply to the medical-pharmaceutical scientists. For example, African-American mistrust of large institutional settings and health and human service agencies is influenced by documented neglect and abuse of human research subjects (Fujimoto 1998; Arean and Gallagher-Thompson 1996). The long history of repression and medical victimization of African-Americans, beginning in the antebellum period (Gamble 1997; King 1997) and culminating in the Tuskegee Syphilis Study (Jones 1992) has contributed to the unwillingness of some African-Americans to participate in health intervention studies.

Green and associates examined perceptions of adults (18 and older) who lived in Jefferson County, Alabama, to determine the effects of the Tuskegee Syphilis Study on African-Americans' willingness to participate in health studies (Green et al. 1997). They found that African-Americans indicated less interest than White Americans in participating in health research or health promotion activities because of the Tuskegee syphilis experiment (22% vs 10%, P<.001), and African-American males reported less interest than White males (27% vs 11%, P<.001). This historical legacy of poor treatment by physicians has major implications on researchers' ability to recruit research participants, especially African-Americans.

Indeed, cases of medical abuse of African-Americans predate the Tuskegee Syphilis Study. Gamble (1997) traced the blatant and racist violations of medical research among African-Americans to the 1800s when Blacks were used as test subjects to promote race-specific stereotypes. A priority goal of such medical research was to provide scientific evidence for widely held beliefs that African-Americans were physically, genetically, and intellectually inferior to Whites. Although these abuses are considered past history, current reported cases of hospitals refusing to provide care to patients (often minority patients) who do not have insurance coverage are often viewed as the continuing legacy of past medical victimization. Communities of color often interpret these current events as validating their belief that the medical establishment (and by extension health researchers) cannot be trusted.

Studies investigating the factors that influence participation and successful community-based interventions among people of color provide additional insight on strategies to remove barriers to participation. In a Heart Health program study targeted at 339 Southeast Asian immigrants, Chen and colleagues (1991) conducted a study to educate this population about cardiovascular risk reduction. Instead of relying on educational print materials, which merely translated information that was not sustainable, their intervention was based on one-on-one counseling and a small group course on healthy cooking. Through this process, the researchers learned that "calendars were very acceptable and attractive to Southeast Asians"; researchers subsequently developed a calendar depicting an identifiable Southeast Asian landmark and displayed a specific heart health education message each month. The researchers also learned through community leaders that video players were popular in 98% of the community's homes and that families often borrowed videos in Southeast Asian languages from neighborhood grocery stores. Through this medium, heart health messages presented by respected community leaders were incorporated into the most popular videos. Failing to sincerely involve community leaders in the planning and implementation of the research is likely to result in limited recruitment and retention of community members in studies.

Factors that may explain the limited participation of African-Americans include lack of understanding of the research study (Coleman et al. 1997), ethnocultural beliefs about the disease or health condition for which the intervention is developed (Erwin et al. 1996), difficulties with transportation to clinic or research site (Smith, Merritt, and Patel 1997), mistrust of health care providers (Green et al. 1997), lack of information about the type of assistance available to facilitate participation (Holder et al. 1998), absence of culturally or racially compatible professional staff (Holder et al. 1998), and limited poststudy interaction with these populations (Coleman et al. 1997). Another factor may be unfamiliarity with research procedures such as randomization, masking, and placebo controls (Fujimoto 1998). The community also may be concerned with sustainability of the care offered through the intervention once the study has ended. It should be noted that many of the barriers to recruiting and retaining people of color in community-based studies apply to the general population as well, particularly among certain socioeconomic classes. Discriminatory practices also lead to marginalization of African-American physicians; they were once excluded from being members of the American Medical Association, and those who were able to obtain their medical education often were denied practicing privileges in many hospitals, and were excluded from scholarly forums (Nickens 1985; Charatz-Litt 1991). Their expertise and recognized presence in the medical community could have prevented some of the suspicion and mistrust of the medical establishment that is now commonplace. The persistent racial disparity in health outcomes and the across-the-board phenomenon of nonparticipation in research efforts makes improving the health status of people of color an urgent priority.

Recruitment Strategies in African-American Communities

While researchers recognize that recruiting ethnically diverse populations may require unique strategies, there is limited evaluation data on which strategies are most effective (Coleman et al. 1997). Documentation of studies that appear to include adequate minority representation often lacks or omits details on recruitment strategies, and this may be the reason that attempts to examine the effectiveness of recruitment methods often lead to inconsistent results. These limitations notwithstanding, results from a few studies offer insights into the usefulness of various recruitment methods. For example, several studies compared passive and active recruitment methods (Coleman et al. 1997; Vogt et al. 1986; Thomas et al. 1994; Wagner et al. 1991). Passive recruitment methods involve eliciting participation in studies through public announcements, for example, on radio and television or in printed communications media such as church bulletins and newspapers. Active recruitment methods involve directly contacting individuals by telephone, by mail, or in person.

Studies that use community recruitment strategies such as radio announcements and public flyers to enroll healthy adults generally yield a low recruitment rate (Holder et al. 1998; Vollmer, Hertert, and Allison 1992). This is particularly true for African-American adults who do not necessarily represent the healthy adult population that is typically recruited for health education intervention research (Jones 1992; Smith, Merritt, and Patel 1997). Recruitment through community outreach is more difficult when researchers do not have established linkages with a recognized local institution. Recruitment becomes harder still when potential participants consider their health status to be too poor for participation in a health study (Flaherty and O'Brien 1992; O'Brien 1983). Another possible factor in limiting an individual's participation may be his/her family's attitudes and beliefs about the health condition being studied. For example, negative feelings may be associated with such conditions as cancer, diabetes, hypertension, and HIV/AIDS (Patrick, Pruchno, and Rose 1998; Fujimoto 1998). Other factors that appear to impede recruitment and retention efforts include negative past experiences with health care providers and the tendency an ill person may have to avoid time commitments that may be required to adhere to a medical regimen, such as commitments that may take time away from the family (Reiss, Gonzalez, and Kramer 1986).

Findings from a study by Coleman and associates (1997) support the need for developing strong relationships with the targeted community. Their study examined efforts to involve a community of older African-Americans in a senior center based health intervention. Focusing on institutions that predominantly served older African-Americans, these researchers employed four recruitment methods: 1) telephone contact (a "phonathon" as well as individual calls made by community board members), 2) printed materials that included a senior center bulletin, community newspaper announcements, and flyers, 3) word of mouth (e.g., friends, family, and outreach workers), and 4) other approaches that included public television announcements and community presentations.

Study results on the number of respondents who learned about the intervention through each recruitment strategy and who later went on to enroll and participate in the study provided useful findings. One hundred seniors heard of the study through telephone contact, and of these, 40% participated. One hundred and four seniors learned about the study through printed material and 38% of them participated. In contrast, 42 seniors learned about the intervention by word of mouth and 74% of them participated. Fourteen seniors learned of the intervention through other approaches (e.g., presentations at the senior center, church presentations, public TV) and 71% of these became participants. Word of mouth was relatively more effective in enrolling participants than either telephone contact (P<.001) or printed materials (P<.001). These findings show that word-of-mouth referrals among individuals who know and trust each other is the most effective recruitment strategy.

This finding also suggests the importance of using direct contact with the community in ways that foster a trusting relationship between researchers and community members. This can be accomplished in several ways: developing an advisory group of community leaders and working closely with social organizations such as the church, fraternal organizations, and athletic groups as well as with medical and educational institutions. Another strategy for gaining trust is for the research team to demonstrate to the community that the research effort will benefit them in other ways (e.g., helping develop a community coalition that can initiate strategies to address other health issues, providing disease-relevant educational programs, providing community services that are not necessarily directly related to the study). The community also needs to know that it will be kept abreast of progress until the research is completed, and that the findings will be presented in a format residents can easily grasp. Finally, the use of focus groups made up of community residents can provide the researchers with useful recruitment and retention information. This interactive process also may provide a foundation of interpersonal connection that is not usually part of the process in randomized, controlled trials. In fact, establishing this connectedness is central to the value of community participation and involvement. It is also central to the value of relationships, kinships, and family in the African-American community.

Health studies that engage families via multisystem approaches have been successful in increasing minority participation. A multisystem approach is anchored in the confluence of social interactions between the family, health care team, and research staff to maximize recruitment and retention (Holder et al. 1998). Focusing on families rather than individuals ensures that valuable information will be obtained on various aspects of disease management, cultural influences, access to health care, familial influence on adoption of health practices, and health-care-seeking behaviors (Young et al. 1996). Studies that focused on children and adolescents in school-based settings have also been shown to be successful in reaching families (Brody, Stoneman, and Gauger 1996; Brody, Arias, and Fincham 1996); a major reason for this success is likely the use of school settings, where there are established communication linkages between school personnel and parents, and recruitment opportunities through these existing organizational structures (e.g., parent-teacher groups, clubs), can be conducted. However, where disconnectedness between parents and schools, such as in some inner-cities, makes school-based strategies unrealistic, a community/parent focused strategy should be employed.

Community Partnership in Health Research

In the last several years, community collaborations have been formed by way of partnerships, consortia, coalitions, and networks to address a myriad of health promotion concerns ranging from tobacco use, substance abuse, and breast cancer to childhood and adult immunizations. Currently, the Centers for Disease Control and Prevention (CDC) and other federal and private organizations are supporting many of these collaborative initiatives with funding, training, and technical assistance (Butterfoss, Goodman, and Wansersman 1996). Strategies focusing on community capacity have been utilized extensively to address outreach and educational efforts, needs assessment initiatives, and planning and implementation of health promotion activities. According to the literature, limited community-capacity strategy related to retention and recruitment of individuals for health research have taken place; however, such efforts are being successfully initiated more often, particularly in recruiting and retaining African-Americans, whose participation in health studies has been limited (Bilworth-Anderson et al. 1993; Thompson et al. 1996). Gorelick and associates (Gorelick et al. 1998) point out that in the African-American community, church leaders, physicians, politicians, civic leaders, the local news media, and "spokesperson celebrities" are credible entities for sanctioning and promoting health initiatives. In this population, initiatives are not likely to be successful without the support of these key community leaders. The researchers further emphasize the importance of including key members of the African-American community in the planning phase as well as supporting the inclusion of community members personally affected by the health concern being addressed. There are initiatives that demonstrate successful community partnerships in research as described in the following projects.

The Detroit Education and Early Detection (DEED) program is a cancer prevention program that has successfully used a community partnership strategy for the recruitment and retention of African-American participants (Parzuchowski et al. 1996). DEED's goal was to develop a model for increasing the participation rates of African-American men in prostate cancer screening efforts. Since its inception in early 1992, DEED has used a community-initiated advisory board made up of local religious, community, and health leaders to guide the research efforts. The advisory board meets twice a month with the DEED team, made up of a program coordinator, a nurse coordinator, a community outreach worker, a clinical team, volunteers, and prostate cancer survivors. Also, every effort is made to hire persons from the community for key positions. DEED's recruitment and retention strategies included outreach and screening efforts after Sunday services, an extensive media campaign, and an educational component. As a result of the "Sunday Service Program," 50% of eligible male church members (aged 40–70 years) took part in the prostate education and screening intervention.

A recruitment and retention effort initiated by Case Western Reserve University and the University Hospital of Cleveland resulted in a marked increase in the number of African-American participants in an Alzheimer's disease research study. The positive outcomes were linked to an extensive community decision-making process and the creation of community recruitment efforts that, via boards, included lay persons affected by the disease (Picot et al. 1996). Since the program's inception, nearly 80% of the subjects returned for follow-up visits, and 15% continued to be assessed by telephone.

In another study focused on caregivers for Alzheimer's disease, Wayne State University researchers found that using a collaborative initiative involving churches and community agencies could improve recruitment and retention of African-American participants (Bilworth-Anderson et al. 1993). Of the 575 family caregivers initially enrolled in the study, 553 (96%) completed a second round of interviews. Completion rates for the 193 African-American participants in the study were similar to those of the White participants. The authors reported that third-round interviews showed similar success.

A fourth initiative with the goal of maximizing the participation of African-Americans was a diabetes study that used a community advisory board to review the survey instrument developed by the research team, identify persons from the community to serve as interviewers, and promote the survey through various community-wide efforts (Burrus, Liburd, Burroughs 1998). Project DIRECT (Diabetes Interventions Reaching and Educating Communities Together) was a community diabetes demonstration project initiated by CDC and the Research Triangle Institute (RTI) with extensive input and ongoing consultation from the community where the project was implemented (Wake County, North Carolina). The overall response rate to the household pilot survey was 77%; of the eligible African-American respondents, 81% completed the household survey and 80% completed a comprehensive medical exam.

Finally, a University of Washington research effort combined several recruitment strategies, including a community-wide approval mechanism, to recruit older African-Americans for a community-based health promotion intervention (Coleman et al. 1997). This initiative focused on nutrition, safety, exercise, and other relevant health topics. The goal of the study was to determine the most effective recruitment strategies for older African-Americans.

In addition to these community-based health promotion interventions, a limited number of projects have been successful in recruiting African-Americans into clinical trials. In a review article titled "Recruiting Minorities into Clinical Trials: Toward a Participant-Friendly System," Swanson and Ward (Swanson and Ward 1995) summarized key issues in the recruitment of racial and ethnic minorities into clinical trials. In addition to addressing recruitment barriers, they identify effective and ineffective methods of recruiting clinical trial participants. Specific community recruitment strategies include developing trust with social organizations, educational institutions, some medical institutions, fraternal organizations, and athletic groups. Other venues include social gatherings such as picnics, political group meetings, and neighborhood improvement groups, which can be used to notify the community about clinical trials in addition to recruiting participants. In order to gain a community's trust, study project staff might participate in volunteer initiatives, conduct educational activities, and work on community-initiated projects, not necessarily linked to the recruitment initiative.

In a study that compares the effect of ethnicity in recruitment into clinical trails, Thompson, Neighbors, Munday, and Jackson (Thompson et al. 1996) successfully recruited African-Americans (compared to their White counterparts) into clinical research at psychiatric hospitals. Four factors were cited for their success: 1) development of a trusting partnership between the researchers and the hospital staff; 2) careful selection of interviewers with experience working in the population and with the health problems; 3) thorough and consistent training sessions for the interviewers including demonstration of an understanding of the survey questionnaire; and 4) addressing cultural sensitivity by matching interviewers with study participants. A second project that successfully recruited African-Americans into a randomized controlled trial is the Cardiovascular Dietary Education System (CARDES) (Kumanyika et al. 1999). CARDES is a cardiovascular nutrition education project for 40–70-year-old, African-American men and women in Washington D.C. Participants were recruited in neighborhood supermarkets for cholesterol and blood pressure screening; screenings were advertised in posters and flyers for "Black men and women concerned about high blood pressure and high cholesterol" and the project identified its affiliation with Howard University.

Researchers across all disciplines should address both historical and current actions and events in minority communities that created an atmosphere of mistrust. Also, the "medical abandonment" of many minority communities has contributed to their limited involvement in determining research agendas (Jack and Liburd 2000). As a result, a tremendous effort will be needed to rebuild trust with minority communities and their recognized local institutions, gatekeepers, and constituents. Re-establishing trust requires considerable human and financial commitments, but most researchers lack resources beyond those required to implement the study protocol. Additionally, most researchers are interested in employing the most effective recruitment methods to obtain an adequate sample size even though they may require less social interaction with minority communities. This approach often creates postrecruitment resentment because community expectations were never addressed and minority participation was limited to "collecting data," with the promise of delivering research findings that would help document the need for additional health services. These services, however, often are never delivered.

Eliminating postrecruitment resentment will require human and fiscal expenditures to engage communities in the often slow and tedious process of communication. Researchers and community must address the nature of the health studies; the benefits of participation; the selection of sites to recruit participants and ways to assist the recruitment process; and the services that will be provided while the health study is being conducted and after data collection results are analyzed. These considerations are important given that traditional methods to recruit minority participants typically do not work (Arean and Gallagher-Thompson 1996), and that recruitment and retention are made easier when methods are tailored to address the issues that prevent potential participants from engaging in research (Burrus, Liburd, and Burroughs 1998).

In general, we propose the following recommendations to encourage the successful use of community capacity-building strategies in recruiting African-Americans for clinical trials and retaining their participation:

- Establish community support well in advance of the research initiative.
- Directly involve community leaders at the onset of the research initiative.
- Provide an opportunity for the community to address concerns about safety and ethical conduct, particularly in light of the past legacy of medical research abuses in minority communities.
- Establish a community advisory committee to develop criteria and strategies and to address ongoing needs of the project.
- Hire a Community Service Coordinator from the community; if money is not available, obtain the services of a committed volunteer who has visibility in the community.
- Establish a community awareness network whose goals are to raise awareness about the study in general and to educate people about the specific health issues being addressed.
- Address the "What's in it for me?" question that can be expected to come from some members of the community.
- Address other barriers to recruitment and retention.

Future Public Health Research and Training in Community-Based Intervention

The difficulty in recruiting and retaining African-Americans as research participants can be addressed by focusing on community-level strategies to involve more African-Americans, on the one hand, and by transforming the way researchers work with African-Americans on the other; most recommendations have emphasized the former—how to involve African-American participants in research. However, a more crucial strategy that is seldom addressed is the need to focus on transforming the practices of public health researchers and scientists so their methodology becomes a facilitator of, rather than a major barrier to, increasing minority participation in studies. As new strategies are developed and proven effective, increasing community participation in research studies, educators should be challenged to simultaneously begin preparing future researchers and health professionals to establish more community-based and culturally based research models. Indeed, strengthening community capacity to increase minority participation in research will become even more important in the future.

Increasingly, researchers and institutions around the world are questioning the serious limitation in focusing on behavior change without giving adequate attention to factors in the social and physical environmental that shape individual roles and expectations and, therefore, health behavior (Institute of Medicine 1994; Rockefeller Foundation 1999; McKinlay and Marceau 1999; Kelly 1999). In fact, many conventional theories and models used to inform public health research and interventions are being challenged for their inadequacy in contexts that are outside the assumptions inherent in these theories and models. Behavior change efforts focus almost exclusively on individuals, and a common assumption is that there is a linear progression from the acquisition of knowledge to a behavioral outcome (Airhihenbuwa and Obregon 2000). Another common value of these classical theories is their search for a single universal solution for all persons regardless of their varied environmental, cultural, or contextual influences. In fact, Cornel West opined that some people are so focused on unlocking the door of opportunity with a single key that in their search for such a door, they pass, unnoticed, many open doors of opportunity (West 1993). This is not to suggest that individuals do not have a crucial role to play in decisions that affect their lives, but rather questions the capacity of individuals to make such decisions without adequate consideration of their community and the broader societal contexts that regulate any available options

Indeed, there are instances when we should focus on individuals, such as when identifying individual researchers with the appropriate methodological experience and background to frame the questions that could lead to the desired health outcome. Such an individual-focused strategy often is not engaged because of the tradition of elevating institutional affiliations (known and familiar institutions) as a higher criterion for funding before individuals. Thus, funding support of research and interventions for addressing health issues is based more on institutional capacity than on individual capacity, both in considering who is to be funded and in selecting the panel that should make the funding decision. Conversely, we focus too much on individuals' health decisions instead of focusing on environmental contexts in terms of factors that shape those decisions.

In response to the need to focus on environmental contexts rather than exclusively on individuals, the Joint United Nations Programme on HIV/AIDS (UNAIDS) recommends that new preventive and educational interventions on HIV/AIDS be focused on five contextual domains that are known to influence behavior outcomes independently or collectively (UNAIDS/Penn State 1999). These domains jointly shape community capacity, which may influence the participation levels of African-Americans in health intervention studies. They are:

- government policy—the role of policy and law in supporting or hindering intervention efforts, e.g., the Tuskegee Syphilis Study;

- social economic status—differential collective or individual income that may allow or prevent adequate intervention, e.g., two individuals with the same income may have different family obligations depending on whether they are first-, second-, or third-generation middle class;

- culture—positive, existential, or negative characteristics that may promote or hinder prevention and care practices, e.g., a culture of collectivism rather than individualism;

- gender relations—status of women in relation to men in society and the community and its influence on sexual negotiation and decision making; and

- spirituality—role of spiritual/religious values in promoting or hindering the translation of prevention, care, and support messages into positive health actions.

Based on these five domains for understanding health behaviors within community and societal contexts, five corresponding professional training domains (Institutional Policy, Social Professional Status, Methodological Culture, Gender Relations and Expectations, and Language and Spirit of Public Health Intervention) are presented for transforming the behaviors of educators and academic institutions. These five domains will be crucial in developing a comprehensive response to the issue of increasing minority participation in health intervention research. They address the training of future public health researchers and practitioners as well as the urgency of bridging the gap in health outcomes between the ethnic minority and the White populations in the U.S. that has become a priority focus of public health interventions. These five domains will be addressed in terms of transforming professorial practices.

Institutional Policy—This is a focus on institutional commitment to community-based strategies. A crucial aspect is the extent to which funding agencies and academic institutions are committed to providing adequate resources for ensuring that a focus on the physical and social environment is a key component of training. An example is the new CDC Racial and Ethnic Approaches to Community Health 2010. In 1998, President Bill Clinton committed the nation to an ambitious goal of eliminating disparities in health status experienced by racial and ethnic minority populations in key areas by the year 2010. In support of this effort, the Department of Health and Human Services identified six priority areas in which racial and ethnic minorities experience serious health disparities. These six priority areas include Infant Mortality, Deficits in Breast and Cervical Cancer Screening and Management, Cardiovascular Disease, Diabetes, Human Immunodeficiency Virus (HIV), Infections/Acquired Immunodeficiency Syndrome (AIDS), and Deficits in Child and/or Adult Immunizations. CDC has awarded several community-based demonstration projects that foster relationships with communities of color and health-related researchers with the goal of reducing health disparities. It is crucial that researchers be adequately rewarded for their contributions and commitment to focusing on community-based strategies.

Social Professional Status—This focuses on the "professorial will" to provide a supportive environment where student training in addressing contextual factors is central to public health research and teaching. This domain can be measured by the number of senior faculty members in an academic unit (department, school, or college) whose research and teaching are focused on this area. Another indicator of social professional status is the proportion of newly hired faculty/staff focusing in this area.

Methodological Culture—This is a focus on methodological approaches and the extent to which the population of interest participates in formulating the research questions. Current approaches largely are based on the individual and familial standards of the majority White population, which has provided most medical research participants in the past. Professional culture can only be understood when methodological approaches engage the population-of-interest as co-researchers. Expanding our current understanding of the role of culture will involve a paradigm shift among health professionals. A critical focus of the new methodological culture is the use of participatory research so that the population of focus becomes a part of the research team. Employing this method promotes ownership of the problems as well as the rewards associated with the research. Addressing cultural sensitivity is an inherent process in participatory research, and contextual strengths and limitations are regularly discussed at project meetings. Another crucial step in transforming the methodological culture is promoting reciprocity in lessons from global interventions. Indeed, much of what has been learned about community-based interventions has come from countries other than the United States. We should acknowledge that globalization makes health intervention lessons a two-way street.

Gender Relations and Expectations—This domain examines the extent to which power relationships, particularly with respect to the role of women in the family, regulate behaviors and places into proper context the practices of targeting women and men in public health interventions (e.g., some women are targeted when men actually are regulating the decisions about sexuality between couples). In this context, human rights and ethics in research should be emphasized. There should be a focus on women's general health as women rather than only as mothers. It also will be useful to prioritize notions of empowerment since the current appropriation is linear (assuming that professionals can empower the disempowered) rather than a robust, collective, and comprehensive evaluation of power relations to ascertain what is possible and practical (Airhihenbuwa 1999).

Language and Spirit of Public Health Intervention—The language of training and exchange is one of the most consistent factors in conditioning a researcher's professional view of how to approach a community. The spirit of the language captures and promotes the values and beliefs of the profession. A major challenge in transforming the methodological approach to professional training in public health is to change professional language that has hitherto described "community" as a problem in need of solution. For example, while the term "community diagnosis" represents the community as a diseased entity, the term "community assessment" encourages us to work with the community itself to recognize its assets (positive), unique identity (existential), and liabilities (negative) (Airhihenbuwa 1999; Green and Kreuter 1999). Other examples of the "language of limitation" include talking about the leading cause of death but not about the leading outcome of life, and discussing "quality of life," which is a somewhat nebulous term that may not be understood in many communities. If in fact the term is understood, communities of color may differ on what the term actually means in their cultural and environmental contexts.

A focus on individuals may condition us to seek self-efficacy, whereas a focus on the physical and social environment of a group should teach us to appreciate community and collective efficacy as advanced by Braithwaite and more recently by Bandura (Bernstein et al. 1994; Bandura 1998). Group and collective efficacy refer to a group's readiness and belief that they are capable of and have the resources to transform the negative health causes and/or outcomes in their environment. A methodological culture that values only what the researcher knows often blames the failure of programs on "cultural barriers" (as though everything cultural is negative), but never credits "cultural strength" for program success (as advanced in the PEN-

3 model) (Airhihenbuwa 1995). Knowledge is not the sole domain of professional institutions, just as belief is not the sole domain of the community. The new professional methodology must recognize the bias inherent in judging knowledge as positive and beliefs as questionable until subjected to the knowledge test. It is time to debunk the notion that knowledge (read: professional values) is a more superior entity than belief (read: community values) when there should not be a hierarchy of importance.

A final aspect of the language of public health is language elasticity. Language elasticity is a term coined by Airhihenbuwa (Airhihenbuwa 1999) to illustrate the importance of recognizing language codes and meanings of different genres. Some languages may be rigid and linear in their application while others are elastic and robust. In developing interventions to modify food practices, a linear and rigid rule in health intervention (as in standard measuring cups for cooking) is important, but equally important and deserving of recognition is an elastic and robust cultural production (as in a pinch or handful). Neither form of measure is superior to the other; they are different and important in their cultural contexts. Indeed, the success of oral rehydration therapy for diarrhea in other countries has been mainly due to the recognition of different ways cultures regulate measurement of food items so that child survival interventions were developed accordingly (Airhihenbuwa 1993). Such success was achieved only by meeting with the people initially and conducting qualitative studies such as focus group interviews to learn about their way of knowing and way of being. Such information may then be incorporated into the research and intervention phase, with members of the community always involved in the planning and implementation process. For example, among African-Americans, levels of physical activity are low even though it is an important intervention for reducing the risk of cardiovascular disease, which is disproportionately high in this group. However, attention to language of intervention will facilitate the promotion of physical activity by stressing leisure-time physical activity, which means the intervention should account for participants' leisure time. Other major considerations found in a focus group study include the time of the day for proposed physical activity, preference for group-based (aerobics, dancing) rather than individual based (jogging, running) activity, and importance of "rest," particularly for the older population and those who have two jobs (Airhihenbuwa et al. 1995).

Conclusion

The most important rule in a community-based research strategy, particularly in clinical trials, is for the researchers to consider the community participants as co-researchers and to consider themselves as co-learners. This new strategy of community-based intervention research, which would maximize the involvement of African-American participants in health and medical research, should begin by transforming the methodological culture of training institutions. Such transformation should prepare students and educators to embrace new professional values and to view the community as an entity with positive, existential, and negative characteristics (Airhihenbuwa 1995;

Airhihenbuwa 1999). It is time for researchers to institutionalize a more comprehensive view that departs from the notion of "diagnosing" communities as if they were problem entities and instead promotes their assets and positive qualities.

References

Airhihenbuwa CO. *Health and Culture: Beyond The Western Paradigm*. Newbury Park, Calif.: Sage Publications, 1995.

Airhihenbuwa C. Health promotion and the discourse on culture: implications for empowerment. *Health Educ Q*. 1994;21:345-353.

Airhihenbuwa CO. Health promotion for child survival in Africa: implications for cultural appropriateness. *Int J Health Educ*. 1993;12(3):10-15.

Airhihenbuwa CO. Of culture and multiverse: renouncing "the universal truth" in health. *J Health Educ*. 1999;30(3):267-273.

Airhihenbuwa CO, Kumanyika S, Agurs TD, Lowe A. Perceptions and Beliefs about Exercise, Rest, and Health among African-Americans. *Am J Health Promotion*. 1995;9(6):426-429.

Airhihenbuwa CO, Obregon R. A critical assessment of Theories/Models used in Health communication for HIV/AIDS. *J Health Commun*. 2000;5:5-15.

Arean PA, Gallagher-Thompson D. Issues and recommendations for the recruitment and retention of older ethnic minority adults into clinical research. *J Consulting Clin Psychol*. 1996; 64(5):875-880.

Asante MK. *The Afrocentric Idea*. Philadelphia, PA: Temple University Press, 1987.

Bandura A. *Social modeling and self-efficacy*. A Report on the Second Conference on Entertainment-Education and Social Change. Baltimore: Johns Hopkins University Center for Communication Programs (JHU/CCP); 1998.

Bernstein E, Wallerstein N, Braithewaite R, Gutierrez L, Labonte R, Zimmerman M. Empowerment forum: a dialogue between guest editorial board members. *Health Educ Q*. 1994;21:281-294.

Bilworth-Anderson P, Burton LM, Johnson LB. Reframing Theories for Understanding Race, Ethnicity, and Families. In: Boss PG, Doherty WJ, LaRossa R, Schumm WR, Steinmets SK, eds. *Sourcebook of Families Theories and Methods: A Contextual Approach*. New York: Plenum Press; 1993;627-646.

Braithwaite RL, Lythcott N. Community empowerment as a strategy for health promotion for black and other minority populations. *JAMA*. 1989;261:282-283.

Braithwaite RL, Taylor SE. *Health Issues in the Black Community*. San Francisco: Jossey-Bass; 1992.

Braslow JT. In the Name of Therapeutics: The Practice of Sterilization in a California State Hospital. *J Hist Med Allied Sci*. 1996;51:29-51.

Brody GH, Arias I, Fincham FD. Linking marital and child attributions to family processes and parent-child relationships. *J Family Psychol*. 1996;10:408-421.

Brody GH, Stoneman Z, Gauger K. Parent-child relationships, family problem-solving behavior, and sibling relationship quality: the moderating role of sibling temperaments. *Child Development*. 1996;67:1289-1300.

Burrus BB, Liburd L, Burroughs A. Maximizing participation by black Americans in population-based diabetes research: The Project DIRECT pilot experience. *J Community Health*. 1998;23(1):15-27.

Butterfoss FD, Goodman RM, Wansersman A. Community coalitions for prevention and health promotion. *Health Educ Res*. 1993;8:315-330.

Butterfoss FD, Goodman RM, Wansersman A. Community coalitions for prevention and health promotion: factors predicting satisfaction, participation, and planning. *Health Educ Q*. 1996;23:65-79.

Chadiha LA, Morrow-Howell N, Darkwa O, McGillick J. Targeting black churches and clergy for disseminating knowledge about Alzheimer's disease and caregiver's support groups. *Am J Alzheimer's Care Related Disord Res*. 1994;May/June:17-20.

Charatz-Litt C. A chronicle of racism: the effects of the white medical community on black health. *J Natl Med Assoc*. 1991;84:17-725.

Chen MS, Kuun P, Guthrie R, Li W, Zaharlick A. Promoting heart health for Southeast Asians: a debate for planning interventions. *Public Health Rep*. 1991;106:304-309.

Coleman EA, Tyll L, LaCroix AZ, et al. Recruiting African American older adults for community-based health promotion intervention: which strategies are effective. *Am J Prev Med.* 1997; 13(6):51-56.

Erwin DO, Spatz TS, Stotts C, Hollenberg JA, Deloney LA. Increasing mammography and breast self-examination in African-American women using Witness Project Model. *J Cancer Educ.* 1996;11(4):210-215.

Flaherty J, O'Brien ME. Family styles of coping in end stage renal disease. *Am Nephrol Nurs Assoc J.* 1992;19:345-350.

Freire P. *Education for Critical Consciousness.* New York: Continuum Press, 1973.

Fujimoto W. Community involvement and minority participation in clinical research. *Diabetes Spectrum.* 1998:11(3);61-165.

Gamble VN. Under the shadow of Tuskegee: African Americans and health care. *Am J Public Health.* 1997;87:1773-1778.

Giroux H A. *Border Crossings: Cultural Workers and the Politics of Education.* New York: Routledge; 1992.

Goodman RM, Speers MA, McLeroy K et al. Identifying and defining the dimensions of community capacity to provide a basis for measurement. *Health Educ Behav.* 1998;25:258-278.

Gorelick P, Harris Y, Burnett B, Bonecutter F. The recruitment triangle: reasons why African Americans enroll, refuse to enroll, or voluntarily withdraw from a clinical trial. *J Natl Med Assoc.* 1998;90:41-145.

Green LW, Kreuter MW. *Health Promotion Planning: An Educational and Ecological Approach,* 3rd ed. Mountain View, California: Mayfield Publishing Company, 1999.

Green LB, Maisiak R, Wang M, Britt MF, Ebeling N. Participation in health education promotion, and health research by African Americans: effects of the Tuskegee Syphilis Experiment. *J Health Educ.* 1997;28:196-201.

Hahn RA. *Sickness and Healing: An Anthropological Perspective.* New Haven, Conn.: Yale University Press, 1995.

Harper, K. *Give Me My Father's Body: The Life of Minik, The New York Eskimo.* South Royalton, Vt.: Steerforth Press, 2000.

Holder B, Turner-Musa J, Kimmel PL, et.al. Engagement of African American families in research on chronic illness: a multisystem recruitment approach. *Family Process.* 1998;37(2):127-151.

Hornblum AM. *Acres of Skin: Human Experiments at Holmesburg Prison.* New York: Routledge; 1998.

Institute of Medicine. Reducing Risks for Mental Disorders: Frontier for Preventive Intervention Research. In: Mrazek PJ, Haggerty RJ, eds; Washington, D.C.: National Academy Press; 1994.

Jack L Jr, Liburd L. Race, ethnicity, and diabetes care: where to from here? *The Diabetes Educator* 2000;26(1):91-93.

Jack L Jr, Liburd L, Vinicor, F, Brody, G, McBride V. The influence of the environmental context on diabetes self-management: a rationale for developing a new research paradigm in diabetes education. *Diabetes Educ.* 1999;25(5):775-790.

Jones KR. Risk of hospitalization for chronic hemodialysis patients. *Image: J Nurs Scholarship.* 1992;24(2):88-94.

Kelly JA. Community-level interventions are needed to prevent new HIV infections. *Am J Public Health.* 1999;89(3):299-301.

King G. The "race" concept in smoking: a review of the research on African Americans. *Soc Sci Med.* 1997;45:1075-1087.

Kumanyika SK, Adams-Campbell L, Van Horn B, et al. Outcomes of a cardiovascular nutrition counseling program in African Americans with elevated blood pressure or cholesterol. *J Am Diet Assoc.* 1999:99(11):1380-1388,1391.

Lupton, D. The Body in Medicine. In *Medicine as Culture: Illness, Disease and the Body in Western Societies.* London: Sage Publications, 1994:20-49.

McKinlay JB, Marceau LD. A tale of 3 tails. *Am J Public Health.* 1999;89(3):295-301.

Nickens HW. A case of professional exclusion in 1870. *JAMA.* 1985;253:2549-2552.

O'Brien ME. *The Courage to Survive: The Life Career of the Chronic Dialysis Patient.* New York: Grune & Statton, 1983.

Parzuchowski J, Gelfand D, Powell I, Cothorn M. Recruitment of African Americans to health care research: lessons from prostate cancer screenings. *J Aging Ethnicity*. 1996;1:27-32.

Patrick JH, Pruchno RA, Rose M. Recruiting research participants: a comparison of the costs and effectiveness of five recruitment strategies. *Gerontologist*. 1998;38(2):295-302.

Picot S, Stuckey J, Smyth K, Whitehouse P. Cultural assessments and the recruitment and retention of African Americans into Alzheimer's disease research. *J Aging Ethnicity*. 1996;1:5-18.

Reiss D, Gonzalez S, Kramer N. Family process, chronic illness, and death. *Arch Gen Psychiatry*. 1986;43:795-804.

Rockefeller Foundation. *Communication for Social Change: A Position Paper and Conference Report*. New York: Rockefeller Foundation; 1999.

Smith ED, Merritt SL, Patel MK. Church-based education: an outreach program for African Americans with hypertension. *Ethnicity Dis*. 1997;2(3):243-253.

Swanson GM, Ward AJ. Recruiting minorities into clinical trails: toward a participant-friendly system. *J Natl Cancer Inst*. 1995;87:1747-1759.

Thomas SB, Quinn SC, Billingsley A, Caldwell C. The characteristics of northern black churches with community health outreach programs. *Am J Public Health*. 1994;84:575-579.

Thompson E, Neighbors H, Munday C, Jackson J. Recruitment and retention of African American patients for clinical trials: an exploration of response rates in an urban psychiatric hospital. *J Consulting Clin Psychol*. 1996;64:861-867.

UNAIDS/Penn State. *Communications Framework for HIV/AIDS: A New Direction*. Airhihenbuwa CO, Makinwa B, Frith M, Obregon R, eds. Geneva, Switzerland: UNAIDS; 1999.

Vogt T, Ireland C, Black D, Camel G, Hughes G. Recruitment of elderly volunteers for a multi-center clinical trial: the SHEP Pilot Study. *Controlled Clin Trials*. 1986;7:118-133.

Vollmer WM, Hertert S, Allison MJ. Recruiting children and their families for clinical trials: a case study. *Controlled Clin Trials* 1992;13:315-320.

Wagner EH, Grothaus LC, Hecht JA, LaCroix AZ. Factors associated with participation in a senior health promotion program. *Gerontologist*. 1991;31:598-602.

West C. *Keeping Faith: Philosophy and Race in America*. Routledge, New York: 1993.

Young R, Edevie S, Young J, Peters J. Issues of recruitment and retention in Alzheimer's research among African and white Americans. *J Aging Ethnicity*. 1996;1:19-25.

Chapter 9

Reflections:
GUIDELINES *for the* INCLUSION *of* WOMEN *and* MINORITIES *in* CLINICAL STUDIES

Judith H. LaRosa, PhD, RN

Introduction

Contrary to an often heard view that ethnic minorities and women have been excluded from biomedical research, they have been included in scientific studies from earliest times in the United States. Indeed, both groups, particularly those who were poor, were research subjects for many scientific studies. They were used, sometimes preferentially, because they often did not understand what participation meant, and if they did not understand, they were often in no position to argue about whether they wished to participate. However, such participation in certain unethical studies during the latter part of the 19th century and into the 20th century (Table 1) stirred public outrage and stimulated important changes in United States public policy, biomedical research, and public perspective. These changes have not been without controversy nor unintended consequences.

This chapter considers some of the issues and events that led to the current federal mandate requiring ethnic minorities and women to be included in clinical studies funded by the National Institutes of Health. It further considers some of the consequences of such legislation.

History: Protectionist Policies 1900-1980

History demonstrates that it takes time for negative social issues to reach public consciousness and concern. History also demonstrates that while concern may exist, a nation must have sufficient resources, social consciousness, and a collective will to bring about positive change.

In the 1800s and early 1900s, a series of health threats emerged and prompted the United States government to initiate protectionist measures in the form of legislation; for example, adulterated foods and medicines were being disseminated widely.

Table 1: Selected Examples of Early Unethical Research

1800s. Sarah Jacobs, known as the Welsh Fasting Girl, was the subject of an experiment in early research on anorexia nervosa. The experiment was apparently quite rigorous, aiming to demonstrate that "no one could live without eating" (Brumberg 1995, Goldstein 1987). She proved that thesis by dying of starvation.

1890s. The practice of oophorectomy, Battey's operation, to "cure" insanity gained a modest following among some gynecologists, especially those associated with state mental institutions. This surgical procedure also offered the opportunity for some clinicians to test their theories of the relationship between insanity and reproductive functions (Scull and Favreau 1986).

1940s. The Nazi medical experiments on unwitting and unwilling prisoners of war are legendary.

1950s. The United States government tested biological warfare weapons on humans. Many of the subjects were 7th Day Adventists in the U.S. Army who volunteered for the tests. Scientists briefed them on the experiments, noted that the biological warfare agents being tested could include Q fever, tularemia, typhoid fever, several types of equine encephalitis, and others. They explained that they could quit at anytime. Inducements were offered for participation (Regis 1999).

1960s. Early experimental birth control medications were tested on poor Puerto Rican women without their consent (Gordon 1990; Reed; Vaughn 1970).

Cocaine was an ingredient of Coca-Cola®; morphine addiction was treated with heroin. As a result, Congress enacted legislation to protect the public through control of the preparation, transportation, and sale of foods and medicines (Food and Drug Administration 2000). Selected examples of such legislation can be found in Table 2.

During the 20th century, biomedical investigation advanced, becoming more sophisticated in design and approach. Clinicians were increasingly aware of the need for research as they sought answers to clinical questions. The public began to view biomedical research as important with the advent of population-protective medications and procedures. For example, antibiotics, which emerged largely during World War II, had a profound effect on reducing battlefield-acquired infections. These medications gradually assumed importance in general medical practice in helping to eradicate any number of bacterial infections. Vaccines to prevent smallpox, polio, and other infectious diseases became universally available. Other scientific advances led to improved disease prevention and treatment.

The public knew that medical advances required experiments, often on human beings, but there was little incentive to participate in such studies. Indeed, many viewed participation in research as something to be avoided (McCarthy 1994), especially given some of the abuses that had occurred. That was underscored at the conclusion of World War II when information came to light of what participation in medical experimentation could mean.

In the mid-1940s evidence of savage human experimentation in Nazi death camps roared forth in the media throughout the world. Physicians and scientists of Hitler's Third Reich conducted these experiments on unwilling and uninformed concentration camp victims. Revelations of these unethical and murderous experiments,

Table 2. Selected Examples of Federal Legislation for Foods and Drugs

1848	Drug Importation Act passed to prevent entry of adulterated drugs into the United States
1902	The Biologics Control Act passed to ensure purity and safety of serums, vaccines, and similar products used to prevent or treat diseases
1906	The Harrison Narcotic Act passed requiring prescriptions for products exceeding the allowable limit of narcotics and mandating increased record-keeping for physicians and pharmacists who dispense narcotics
1927	Food, Drug, and Insecticide Administration assumed regulatory functions. The name changed to Food and Drug Administration in 1930
1938	Federal Food, Drug, and Cosmetic Act enacted, encompassing a range of provisions relating to food and drug safety

(http://www.fda.gov/backgrounders/miles.html)

revealed during the Nuremberg War Crimes Trials, shocked the world. At the conclusion of the trials, the Nuremberg War Crimes court released the Nuremberg Code of Ethics—a document delineating ethical action on the inclusions of participants in studies (McCarthy 1994). Governments and organizations in a number of countries, including the United Nations gathered to consider how to prevent such atrocities from ever occurring again. Chapter 3 in this volume, by Heitman and Wells, provides a detailed examination of the unethical treatment of individuals in the realm of medical research.

After World War II, the economy advanced and the affordability of radio and television meant that most homes could now have access to global information. Americans settled into a strong belief in the "American Way." Many now had sufficient resources, social consciousness, and collective will to effect change. Table 3 reflects some of the landmark events dedicated to the protection of human rights that emerged following World War II.

Over the space of two decades, medical, ethical, and legal experts created guidelines that would, they hoped, forever circumscribe what could and could not ethically occur in medical experimentation using human beings. One of the most compelling and instructive of these documents was the *Belmont Report* released in 1978 (National Commission for the Protection of Human Subjects of Biomedical and Behavioral Research 1978). This report identified three principles required of the individual or organization including humans in biomedical and behavioral research:

Respect for persons—requires that each individual must be regarded as autonomous and those who are not (vulnerable populations) should be given special attention and protection,

Beneficence—requires that benefits must be maximized and risk minimized, and

Justice—requires that individuals participating in such research must be selected fairly.

These three principles have served as the basis for inclusion of individuals in biomedical and behavioral research studies and were incorporated into federal regulations during the 1970s.

Table 3. Selected International and National Protectionist Policies for Humans Involved in Biomedical Research *(McCarthy 1994)*

1946-47	Nuremberg War Crimes Trials—Nuremberg Code of Ethics
1950	United Nations Declaration of Human Rights
1966	U.S. Public Health Service Policy and Procedures Order 129—Policy on the Protection of Human Subjects; Revised in 1967 and 1969
1971	U.S. Department of Health, Education, and Welfare policy on the protection of human subjects promulgated
1974	U.S. Department of Health, Education, and Welfare issues policy on the protection of human subjects in research—45 CFR 46. Similar to the previous protectionist policies, but more stringent.
	National Commission for the Protection of Human Subjects of Biomedical and Behavioral Research (The Commission) formed. Recommends more stringent protectionist policies.
	Institutional Review Boards required at research institutions
1977	Food and Drug Administration prohibits women of childbearing age and pregnant women from participating in Phase I trials
1978	The Commission releases the *Belmont Report*, which delineates three ethical principles

But new evidence came to light during the 1970s that provoked further concern on inclusion of humans in biomedical research. Americans were shocked to learn that their own federal government, the United States Public Health Service, had allowed another medical experimentation outrage—The Tuskegee Syphilis Study (Table 4). Not only did this study and ensuing events further underscore the need for strong and enforceable national ethics policies in research, but it confirmed to many African-Americans that once again they were being treated very differently. Other findings released during this period further focused attention on the need for even more stringent protectionist policies.

- 1963. Individuals in the Jewish Chronic Disease Hospital in Brooklyn were given live cancer cells for the purpose of examining the immune system and cancer. No informed consent was obtained (Faden and Beauchamp, 1986).

- The acceptance that the nonsteroidal estrogen-like compound diethylstilbestrol (DES), originally viewed as a therapeutic breakthrough to women threatening to miscarry, was, in fact, a carcinogen (NIH 1992).

These events had a profound effect on the participation of ethnic minorities and women in studies. Regulation 45 CFR 46 was created to protect individuals from participating in studies who have not been fully informed of what they are being asked to do and agree to the tasks required of them. Thus, individuals cannot be legally coerced into another Tuskegee-like study.

Restrictions were particularly stringent for pregnant women. For example, in 1975 the Department of Health and Human Services regulation (45 CFR 46) stated that pregnant women should be viewed as part of "vulnerable" populations; they cannot

Table 4. Tuskeegee Syphilis Study: 1932–1972

The Study of Untreated Syphilis in the Negro Male

Purpose: To study the long-term effects of untreated syphilis in African-American men

Subjects: 600 African-American men—399 in the experimental group and 201 in the control group

Place: Macon County, Alabama. Subsequently included Albemarle County, Virginia; Glynn County, Georgia; Pitt County, North Carolina; Tipton County, Tennessee (Jones 1981)

Informed Consent: None. Participants were offered a number of incentives: free transportation to/from clinic, meals on visit days, free physicals, some free medical treatment, free burial. Participants were not informed that they had syphilis, merely "bad blood."

Sponsor: United States Public Health Service (USPHS)

Participant Institution: Tuskeegee Institute. Tuskeegee was able to benefit through internship training and employment for nurses

Outcome: With the advent of penicillin, a treatment for syphilis, participants were not informed; in fact, every effort was made to avoid informing and deny treatment. The USPHS and local physicians and health departments joined forces to keep patients from treatment

(http://members.com/jtstocks/prof/ethnics/tuskg.html; http://www.dc.peachnet.edu).

be assumed capable of determining whether they should participate in studies. In 1977, the Food and Drug Administration followed suit and restricted the participation of women of childbearing potential in all early (Phase I) drug trial studies with the exception of life-threatening situations.

During the 1950s and 1960s, biomedical research study designs became even more sophisticated and advanced. Clinical trials, the "gold standard" of clinical studies, emerged as an important asset in clinical research.

Certain design principles became firmly entrenched in the research community. For example, study design requires minimizing external threats to validity, and as such, scientists seek participants who will remain as stable as possible during the testing and have few mitigating factors that would influence the disease, disorder, or condition under study. Pre- and postmenopausal women clearly present a problem in such designs. Premenopausal women cycle hormonally, thereby creating unwanted variation. Postmenopausal women have ceased to cycle but are still different from men and premenopausal women. Ethnic minorities present a problem in that they might introduce a genetic difference or cultural bias into the study design.

The issue of recruitment and retention of study participants also present problems. Recruitment and retention can require substantial costs. Thus, scientists sought the least difficult methods of attracting and retaining individuals. Potential participants who have significant barriers to participation (transportation, family obligations, time constraints, different language, and other issues) were to be avoided. Finally, ethnic minority groups, particularly African-Americans who have a long history of abuse by the research community, were, and continue to be, understandably reluctant to participate in biomedical research studies (Savitt 1982; Byrd and Clayton 1992).

Thus, prior to 1993 scientists generally sought White men, the preponderance of males in the United States, as study participants. They were the easiest to include into studies. They do not cycle; they remain relatively constant throughout a life-time—or so many scientists have presumed—and they are in ample supply. This resulted in a dearth of information regarding women and minorities across a wide spectrum of diseases, disorders, and conditions that affected them.

The effect of these regulations, created prior to 1993, has been both positive and negative. On the positive side, they have created an environment in which scien-tists must ensure that each study participant understands what she or he is being asked to do and agrees to participate with that knowledge and without coercion. Vulnerable populations must be protected and all studies must be reviewed and vet-ted by external review groups.

On the negative side, the regulations have created restrictions on who can par-ticipate, even knowledgeably and willingly. For example, until the last few years, women of childbearing age and pregnant women have had their rights abridged because they were defined by law as "vulnerable" and therefore not autonomous—incapable of making an informed decision. The rationale was that if a woman became pregnant, her participation in the study might create teratogenic effects in her unborn child. As such, the very possibility that she might become pregnant not only barred her from participation but also barred her from deciding whether she wished to par-ticipate. However, many women of this age group have no intention of becoming pregnant nor would be in a situation in which they might. Therefore, to prohibit them from making an informed decision about participating abridges their rights.

History: Addressing the Inequities 1980–2000

These different regulations, designed to protect individuals, created unintended con-sequences. Review of the scientific literature from the late 1960s until recently shows that substantial biomedical information has been lacking across the sexes and eth-nic minority groups. Selected examples follow.

- Women may respond differently to diseases, disorders, and conditions than do men. For example, women and men may present differently with a myocardial infarction; with osteoporosis; with breast cancer. Why?

- Women of different racial and ethnic groups appear to develop diseases, dis-orders, and conditions at different ages. For example, White and Asian women tend to develop osteoporosis proximal to their menopause, while African-American women are more susceptible later in life. Why?

- Members of different racial and ethnic groups may respond differently to med-ications and procedures. For example, African-Americans respond differently to certain hypertensive medications than do Whites. Why?

These are well-known examples of questions that have not yet been fully answered. Clearly, questions remain as to what other differences and similarities exist and what their implications are for clinical application.

In the 1980s, scientists and clinicians, women's health advocates, and policy makers, realizing this deficit in sex and ethnic minority biomedical data, began to push for increased attention to studies on ethnic minorities and women. By the mid-1980s federal interest was sufficient to focus attention on this lack of information. The concept that "one size does not fit all"—that biomedical study findings on White males are not universally applicable to women and minorities—was finally acknowledged. Furthermore, it was acknowledged that while protectionist policies are vital, they should not to be used to exclude ethnic minorities and women from studies.

A number of events occurred that propelled ethnic minority and women's health forward nationally. In 1990, the National Institutes of Health created two new offices within the Office of the Director of NIH: The Office of Research on Minority Health and the Office of Research on Women's Health. Other federal agencies followed suit. Health advocates—The Society for the Advancement of Women's Health Research, ACT-UP, the Breast Cancer Coalition, and others—lobbied Congress intensively for increased funding for their particular cause.

In 1993, Congress enacted legislation, Public Law 103-43 (The NIH Revitalization Act of 1993) that officially established the Office of Research on Minority Health and the Office of Research on Women's Health and mandated the inclusion of women and minorities in clinical studies supported by the NIH. This legislation was set against the earlier legislation that mandated the ethical treatment of individuals participating in such studies. Table 5 presents a brief history of the events that led to the federal legislation mandating the inclusion of women and minorities in clinical studies.

The National Institutes of Health Revitalization Act of 1993 required that the National Institutes of Health must:

- ensure that women and members of minority groups and their subpopulations are included in all human subject research;
- for Phase III clinical trials, ensure that women and minorities and their subpopulations are included such that valid analysis of differences in intervention effect can be accomplished;
- not allow cost as an acceptable reason for excluding these groups; and
- initiate programs and support for outreach efforts to recruit these groups into clinical studies.

In response to this mandate, the NIH created the *NIH Guidelines on the Inclusion of Women and Minorities as Subjects in Clinical Research*, crafted the *National Institutes of Health Outreach Notebook for the NIH Guidelines on the Inclusion of Women and Minorities as Subjects in Clinical Research*, and conducted a series of workshops throughout the scientific community to educate regarding the guidelines. Similarly, other groups—the then Office of Protection from Research Risks (OPRR), Public Responsibility in Medicine and Research (PRIM&R), and local institutions—provided similar fora for education and discussion.

Yet, despite documented need for such inclusion, there was still an outcry against such governmental intervention. Some noted that it was creating a quota system; others believed that it would create such a monetary burden that funding would be

Table 5. A Selected History of Women's Health: 1974–1994

1974	• Congressional Caucus for Women's Issues formed
1986	• *Report of the Public Health Task Force on Women's Health Issues*
	• NIH Guidelines on the Inclusion of Women in Clinical Studies
1988	• Government Accounting Office Report: *Problems Implementing Policy on Women in Study Populations*
1990	• Office of Research on Women's Health established at NIH
	• NIH Guidelines on the Inclusion of Minorities and Women in Study Populations
	• Office of Women's Health, Alcohol, Drug Abuse, and Mental Health Administration (ADAMHA)
1991	• National Conference sponsored by ORWH, NIH: *Opportunities for Research on Women's Health*
	• *Journal of Women's Health* created
	• First woman director of NIH appointed: Bernadine Healy, MD
	• Antonio Novello, MD, a pediatrician, is named Surgeon General of the United States
	• The Women's Health Initiative, the largest preventive clinical trial ever mounted, is initiated to study prevention in postmenopausal women through lifestyle modification for heart disease, cancer, and osteoporosis. The study will recruit over 100,000 post-menopausal women.
1992	• Called by many in the media the "Year of the Women"
	• National Conference sponsored by ORWH, NIH: *Women in Biomedical Careers: Dynamics of Changes, Strategies for the 21st Century*
	• Society for the Advancement of Research on Women's Health sponsors first annual Congress on Women's Health in Washington, D.C.
1993	• Jocelyn Elders, MD, a pediatrician, is named Surgeon General of the United States
	• Office of Research sponsored by Women's Health, NIH, and Office of Women's Health, SAMHSA, mandated in legislation
	• Department of Defense was directed to provide $212 million from its budget for breast cancer research and to initiate an office of women's health
	• Congress mandates inclusion of women and minorities as subjects in clinical research supported by NIH
	• National Conference sponsored by ORWH, NIH: *Recruitment and Retention of Women in Clinical Studies*
	• Breast Cancer Coalition delivered over 3 million signatures to President Clinton urging further and directed efforts in breast cancer research and led to the National Breast Cancer Action Plan in 1993
1994	• First congressionally mandated guidelines to include women in biomedical research issued by NIH
	• National Academy of Sciences/Institute of Medicine released *Women and Health Research: Ethical and Legal Issues of Including Women in Clinical Studies*
	• Department of Health and Human Services Breast Cancer Action Plan implemented for research and treatment nationally
	• November elections: Congress rescinds funding support for Congressional Caucus for Women's Issues and other special caucuses; funding for scientific research at risk with budget balancing efforts on Capitol Hill

limited to a few grand studies (Meinert 1995; Piantadosi and Wittes 1993; Marshall 1994; Satel 1995; Charrow 1994; Wechsler 1993.) Alternately, others believed that it was a positive intervention and the ensuing data would enhance clinical interventions and direct further research. (Watanabe 1995; Walker 1996; Freedman, Simon et al. 1995).

A review of NIH research funding since the implementation of the legislation and guidelines clearly reveals such legislation has not halted scientific advances nor relegated research studies to a few large-scale trials. Indeed, they have expanded the scope of research and provided even more information. Scientific inquiry has continued its advances and provides even more specific information for targeted clinical interventions and more refined research.

A FY2003 *Computer Retrieval of Information on Scientific Projects* (CRISP) review using the term "minority" produced 2,244 results, including

- Cultural Perspectives on Minority Identity
- Measuring Sexual Minority Status Among Women Drug Users
- Culturally Focused Skills Training for Native Children to Enhance Self Concept
- Physical Activity Assessment in Multi-Ethnic Women
- Minority Alcohol Use/Abuse—Protective and Risk Factors
- Culturally Appropriate Program to Prevent Substance Use Among Latino Adolescents
- Managed Care's Impact on Minority Physicians and Patients
- Cultural Responses to Illness in Minority Aged
- Ethnic Differences in Adolescents' Mental Distress
- Mental Illness in Super-Maximum Security Prison Units: B
- Brief Intervention to Reduce Injury in Minorities

To review studies funded by the NIH, consult the NIH website (http://www.nih. gov/CRISP). Federal, state, and local governments, as well as other organizations, are now actively supporting and engaged in research examining racial/ethnic differences.

In 1994, NIH initiated a computerized track system to monitor and evaluate the changes brought about by this new mandate. In 2002, a new system was implemented that streamlines the process of accruing and managing the data, meeting the revised forms and data collection formats, and enhances reporting to the various agencies requiring the information. The system continues to be modified as needed. In addition, the NIH provides necessary educational training sessions, information materials, and resources to guide NIH employees, scientists, and clinicians in the myriad issues surrounding the recruitment and retention of individuals in studies and management of data (NIH 2000).

Women and minorities are now systematically included in NIH-funded research. (NIH Implementation of the NIH Guidelines Comprehensive Report 2000a). NIH tracking system reports from 1995 to 2002 can be found on the Office of Research on Women's Health website: www.nih.gov/orwh/inclusion.html. Tables 5–7 present selected data from NIH extramural funding from FY 2000 to 2002—the latest report available (NIH/ORWH 2003). A note of caution in interpreting the tables is warranted. The NIH does not insist on inclusion of women and minorities based on census track figures. Rather, the scientific question and incidence/prevalence of the disease in different populations drives the recruitment of individuals into studies. For example, the Women's Health Initiative, a set of ongoing 10-year clinical studies of over 100,000 postmenopausal women, added significantly to the numbers of women enrolled in NIH-funded studies. There is no comparable large-scale study currently underway in men. Some examples of single-sex studies follow.

Males Only

Osteoporotic Fractures in Men
Molecular Epidemiology of Testicular Carcinoma
The Biological Basis of Alcohol-Induced Brain Damage

Females Only

Risk Factors for Physical Disability in Aging Women
Effects of Partner Violence Victimization in Drug Use
Pathogenesis of Health Disparities in Pre-Term Birth

Single-sex studies or studies affecting a particular racial or ethnic group are certainly warranted. However, each NIH institute or center must maintain a balanced sex and racial/ethnic profile in its studies.

Table 6 presents data on the level of compliance on extramural applications from 2000–2002. Clearly, the number of unacceptable applications remains fairly constant for both minorities and women. For example, the percentage of applications with unacceptable minority inclusion varied between 2.18% and 2.57% in 2000–2002. Data from FY 1995 show that the percentage was 3.43%. Similarly, the number of applications with unacceptable sex/gender inclusion was 0.57% in January 2000 and 0.50% in October 2002. In January 1995, the number was 0.65%. Overall, the number of applications with unacceptable inclusion for both women and minorities remains small and relatively constant.

Table 7 examines the "bars-to-funding" and resolutions that occurred during FY 2000–2002. As noted in the federal law, PL 103-43, the NIH cannot fund research that does not meet the specifications of inclusion. In the period 2000–2002, the percentage of awards that met the requirements ranged from 96% to 97%. However, in some instances the initial application did not meet the requirements. Table 6 indicates where the bar-to-funding was lifted when NIH program staff deemed that the applicants had:

- provided additional information showing that the criteria for inclusion had been met;
- modified the study design to meet the inclusion criteria;
- corrected errors in initial coding of subjects in the proposed study; or
- determined that other factors were operating, i.e., there was an existing cohort, tissue specimens were unidentified, or records were unavailable.

Table 6. Level of Compliance with Inclusion Policy in New Extramural Grant Applications as Assessed During Scientific Peer Review for the Fiscal Period 2000–2002

Council Dates:	Jan-00	May-00	Aug-00	Oct-00	Jan-01	May-01	Aug-01	Oct-01	Jan-02	May-02	Aug-02	Oct-02
Total number of applications reviewed	13,195	14,967	906	13,716	13,521	14,419	917	14,277	14,372	16,023	1,370	16,868
Number of applications with human subjects	5,255	6,160	406	5,772	5,512	6,068	585	5,936	5,836	6,895	733	7,009
Number (percent) of applications approved by IRG as submitted	4,967 (94.51)	5,825 (94.56)	390 (96.05)	5,465 (94.68)	5,244 (95.14)	5,702 (93.97)	562 (96.07)	5,559 (93.65)	5,446 (93.32)	6,448 (93.52)	683 (93.18)	6,556 (93.54)
Number (percent) of applications with unacceptable *minority-only* inclusion	115 (2.18)	119 (1.93)	8 (1.97)	112 (1.94)	99 (1.80)	143 (2.36)	5 (0.85)	142 (2.39)	168 (2.88)	163 (2.36)	21 (2.86)	180 (2.57)
Number (percent) of applications with unacceptable *sex/gender-only* inclusion	30 (0.57)	25 (0.40)	0 (0.00)	28 (0.48)	14 (0.25)	29 (0.48)	6 (1.03)	23 (0.39)	31 (0.53)	30 (0.44)	1 (0.14)	35 (0.50)
Number (percent) of applications with both unacceptable *minority* **and** *sex/gender* inclusion	143 (2.72)	191 (3.10)	16 (3.94)	167 (2.89)	155 (2.81)	194 (3.20)	12 (2.05)	212 (3.57)	191 (3.27)	254 (3.68)	28 (3.82)	238 (3.40)
Total number (percent) of applications with unacceptable *minority* inclusion	258 (4.90)	310 (5.03)	16 (3.94)	279 (4.83)	254 (4.61)	337 (5.55)	17 (2.91)	354 (5.96)	359 (6.15)	417 (6.05)	49 (6.68)	418 (5.96)
Total number (percent) of applications with unacceptable *sex/gender* inclusion	173 (3.29)	216 (3.51)	8 (1.97)	195 (3.38)	169 (3.07)	223 (3.68)	18 (3.08)	235 (3.96)	222 (3.80)	284 (4.12)	29 (3.96)	273 (3.89)
Total number (percent) unacceptable applications as submitted	288 (5.48)	335 (5.44)	16 (3.94)	307 (5.32)	268 (4.86)	366 (6.03)	23 (3.93)	377 (6.35)	390 (6.68)	447 (6.48)	50 (6.82)	453 (6.46)

Table 7. Extramural Research Awards Funded for the Fiscal Period 2000–2002: Bars-to-Funding and Resolutions

Council Dates:	Jan-00	May-00	Aug-00	Oct-00	Jan-01	May-01	Aug-01	Oct-01	Jan-02	May-02	Aug-02	Oct-02
Total number of awards	4,415	4,960	307	4,389	4,441	4,892	348	4,495	4,480	5,058	390	3,707
Number of awards involving human subjects	1,633	1,964	129	1,683	1,649	1,896	200	1,697	1,676	2,022	215	1,319
Number (percent) of awards involving human subjects that met the inclusion requirements as submitted	1,582 (96.87)	1,893 (96.38)	124 (96.12)	1,632 (96.96)	1,599 (96.97)	1,821 (96.04)	188 (94.00)	1,644 (96.88)	1,625 (96.96)	1,947 (96.29)	202 (93.95)	1,284 (97.35)
Number (percent) of awards where *minority-only* bar-to-funding was removed by program staff (M_U)	18 (1.10)	27 (1.37)	1 (0.77)	23 (1.36)	18 (1.09)	25 (1.32)	7 (3.50)	26 (1.53)	19 (1.13)	31 (1.53)	3 (1.40)	15 (1.14)
Number (percent) of awards where *sex/gender-only* bar-to-funding was removed by program staff (G_U)	13 (0.79)	7 (0.35)	0 (0.00)	8 (0.47)	4 (0.24)	3 (0.16)	0 (0.00)	4 (0.24)	5 (0.30)	6 (0.30)	0 (0.00)	7 (0.53)
Number (percent) of awards where both *minority* **and** *sex/gender* bar-to-funding were removed by program staff	20 (1.22)	37 (1.88)	4 (3.10)	20 (1.18)	28 (1.70)	47 (2.48)	5 (2.50)	23 (1.36)	27 (1.61)	38 (1.88)	10 (4.65)	13 (0.99)
Total number (percent) of awards where *minority* bar-to-funding was removed by program staff	38 (2.32)	64 (3.25)	5 (3.87)	43 (2.55)	46 (2.79)	72 (3.80)	12 (6.00)	49 (2.89)	46 (2.74)	69 (3.41)	13 (6.05)	28 (2.12)
Total number (percent) of awards where *sex/gender* bar-to-funding was removed by program staff	33 (2.02)	44 (2.24)	4 (3.10)	28 (1.66)	32 (1.94)	50 (2.64)	5 (2.50)	27 (1.59)	32 (1.91)	44 (2.18)	10 (4.65)	20 (1.52)
Total number (percent) of awards where bar-to-funding was removed	51 (3.12)	71 (3.61)	5 (3.87)	351 (3.03)	50 (3.03)	75 (3.96)	12 (6.00)	53 (3.12)	51 (3.04)	75 (3.71)	13 (6.05)	35 (2.65)

Table 8 presents the total enrollment for all NIH extramural research protocols funded in FY 2001 and reported in 2002. Please note that the new racial/ethnic codes are now in use. Among the racial/ethnic groups the highest enrollment occurs among Whites, at 60%, and the lowest among American Indians and Alaskan Natives, 1.7%. Among the designated minority groups, Blacks represent 12% of the enrolled study participants, followed by Asians at 8%, Hispanics or Latinos at 6.6%, and Hawaiian/Pacific Islander at less than 1%. Individuals reporting more than one race represented less than 1% and those reporting Unknown represented 16%. As shown in previous NIH inclusion data, females substantially outnumber males in studies— 68% vs 31% respectively in 2001. While there were more females than males in studies overall, this difference did not exist across the different racial/ethnic groups.

Table 9 presents the male- and female-only studies funded in 2001 and reported in 2002. When the data are examined this way, the female:male ratio is less disparate, 52.4% vs 45.7%, respectively, than when considered in the aggregate.

Reflections

What is clear is that the guidelines have had an overall positive effect for both women and minorities. A brief review of the literature in the past five years indicates that studies exist comparing males and females across racial/ethnic lines. These data are now available to clinicians for adoption into practice and to scientists for further research.

Women's centers have sprung up across the country with a focus on inclusiveness across ages and racial/ethnic groups. While many of the centers still focus on reproductive health, increasing numbers are directing their services to the totality of women's health needs. Attention to racial and ethnic differences is usually integrated into those services. Urban and rural community organizations direct attention to women's health efforts in an effort to drive knowledge and prevention efforts firmly into community action. These organizations increasingly integrate scientific and cultural information into material and programs for the populations that they serve.

Congress and other policy makers are now more aware of the need for equity in biomedical and behavioral research. That awareness has been reflected in funding streams for specific diseases and programs.

One of the more recent and exciting advances was the recent legislation, *Minority Health in Health Disparities Research and Education Act of 2000*. This act (Public Law [PL] 106-525) passed in the 106th Congress on November 26, 2000. The act mandates that the NIH Office of Research on Minority Health advance to NIH Center status, now known as the National Center on Minority Health and Health Disparities. The advancement to center status at NIH means that that center can fund biomedical research studies directly. Heretofore, the Office of Research on Minority Health had to fund all of its studies in collaboration with other NIH institutes and centers. The new National Center on Minority Health and Health Disparities is able to direct and fund its own studies.

Public and patient awareness has been heightened. Companies and media address issues of women's and minority health regularly. Websites have sprung up.

Table 8. Aggregate Enrollment Data for All Extramural Research Protocols Funded in FY 2001 and Reported in FY 2002

Total Number (%) of All Subjects by Race

	AI/AN	Asian	Black	Hawaiian/PI	White	More than One Race	Other & Unknown	Total
Female	51,173 (1.55)	271,731 (8.21)	371,468 (11.22)	8,554 (0.26)	1,946,559 (58.81)	18,376 (0.56)	641,925 (19.39)	3,309,786 (75.15)
Male	26,272 (2.49)	79,857 (7.57)	168,857 (16.00)	7,981 (0.76)	698,010 (66.15)	12,267 (1.16)	62,019 (5.88)	1,055,263 (23.96)
Unknown	289 (0.74)	2,461 (6.31)	7,451 (19.10)	5,101 (13.08)	6,972 (17.88)	312 (0.80)	16,418 (42.09)	39,004 (0.89)
Total	77,734 (1.77)	354,049 (8.04)	547,776 (12.44)	21,636 (0.49)	2,651,541 (60.21)	30,955 (0.70)	720,362 (16.36)	4,404,053 (100.00)

Female	6,238,525 (68.12)		Male	2,855,387 (31.18)	Unknown	64,859 (0.71)	Total	9,158,771 (100.00)

Total Number (%) of All Subjects by Ethnicities

	Not Hispanic	Hispanic or Latino	Unknown/Not Reported	Total
Female	2,237,035 (67.59)	208,844 (6.31)	863,907 (26.10)	3,309,786 (75.15)
Male	813,756 (77.11)	81,853 (7.76)	159,654 (15.13)	1,055,263 (23.96)
Unknown	21,161 (54.25)	1,732 (4.44)	16,111 (41.31)	39,004 (0.89)
Total	3,071,952 (69.75)	292,429 (6.64)	1,039,672 (23.61)	4,404,053 (100.00)

Number of protocols with enrollment data: 2,758.
AI/AN = American Indian/Alaska Native; PI = Pacific Islander.

Table 9. Aggregate Enrollment Data for Extramural Research Protocols Excluding Male-Only and Female-Only Protocols, Funded in FY 2001 and Reported in FY 2002

Total Number (%) of All Subjects by Race

	AI/AN	Asian	Black	Hawaiian/PI	White	More than One Race	Other & Unknown	Total
Female	27,471 (2.38)	73,888 (6.40)	199,564 (17.29)	8,231 (0.71)	745,791 (64.62)	12,665 (1.10)	86,501 (7.50)	1,154,111 (52.47)
Male	26,096 (2.59)	75,650 (7.52)	162,359 (16.13)	7,958 (0.79)	664,642 (66.04)	11,541 (1.15)	58,129 (5.78)	1,006,375 (45.75)
Unknown	289 (0.74)	2,461 (6.31)	7,451 (19.10)	5,101 (13.08)	6,972 (17.88)	312 (0.80)	16,418 (42.09)	39,004 (1.77)
Total	53,856 (2.45)	151,999 (6.91)	369,374 (16.79)	21,290 (0.97)	1,417,405 (64.44)	24,518 (1.11)	161,048 (7.32)	2,199,490 (100.00)

Female	2,859,832 (50.65)		Male	2,721,783 (48.20)	Unknown	64,859 (0.71)	Total	5,646,474 (100.00)

Total Number (%) of All Subjects by Ethnicities

	Not Hispanic	Hispanic or Latino	Unknown/Not Reported	Total
Female	805,206 (69.77)	86,756 (7.52)	262,149 (22.71)	1,154,111 (52.47)
Male	774,209 (76.93)	79,388 (7.89)	152,778 (15.18)	1,006,375 (45.75)
Unknown	21,161 (54.25)	1,732 (4.44)	16,111 (41.31)	39,004 (1.77)
Total	1,600,576 (72.77)	167,876 (7.63)	431,038 (19.60)	2,199,490 (100.00)

Number of protocols with enrollment data: 2,266.
AI/AN = American Indian/Alaska Native; PI = Pacific Islander.

Yet, 10 years after the implementation of these regulations, one must consider whether what has been done is sufficient and whether any unintended consequences have resulted. Two major issues arise for further consideration, especially as they apply to ethnic minority populations.

* What about the apparent funding inequity between the sexes?
* What about the disparities in the inclusion of different racial/ethnic groups?

Women vs Men. Men now represent a smaller population being studied by NIH-funded scientists, and men-only studies are fewer. Is that because men's health is now less important? Is it that there are fewer large-scale single-sex studies, such as the Women's Health Initiative, being conducted in men? Is this an overcorrection for equity? If so, why?

A men's health equity movement has arisen. Advocates, concerned that U.S. men die an average of seven years earlier than women and continue to suffer diseases that, as yet, do not have assured cures, are fostering men's health programs and centers. Websites that cater specifically to men's health are available, and increasing numbers of television and radio shows feature men's health programming.

These concerns, as well as scientific curiosity about the differences between men and women, have given rise to requests for action. A number of scientists, both male and female, have advocated research examining sex and gender differences in health and disease. The 1999 ORWH report, *Agenda for Research on Women's Health for the 21st Century*, has a section devoted to sex and gender differences and the need for such research. The Society for the Advancement of Women's Health Research has actively promoted the study of sex/gender differences.

In 1999, several organizations[1] came together and commissioned a study from the National Academy of Sciences Institute of Medicine: *Exploring the Biological Contributions to Human Health: Does Sex Matter?* (IOM 2001). The multidisciplinary team of women and men prepared an exciting and scientifically provocative report that has already contributed to heightened interest and funding in the research community. The summary of the report states:

> Despite the progress made in focusing on women's health research and including women in clinical trials, such research will have limited value unless the underlying implications—that is, the actual differences between males and females that make such research so critical—are systematically studied and elucidated. Such research can enhance the basis for interpreting the results of separate studies with males and females, helping to clarify findings of no essential sex differences and suggesting mechanisms to be pursued when sex differences are found. (IOM 2001)

A *Computer Retrieval of Information on Scientific Projects* (CRISP) review of FY 2003 NIH funded research using the terms "sex" and "gender" produced 3,438 "hits" (http://www.nih.gov/CRISP) and included studies such as:

---

[1] DHHS Office of Women's Health, NIH Office of Research on Women's Health, National Institute of Environmental Health Sciences, National Institute on Drug Abuse, Food and Drug Administration, Environmental Protection Agency, National Aeronautics and Space Administration, Society for Women's Health Research, Research Foundation for Health and Environmental Effects, Ortho-McNeil/Johnson & Johnson, and Unilever United States Foundation.

- Gender Differences in Drug Abuse
- Gender, Power, and Suseptibility to STDS/HIV in India
- Sex Differences in Inflammatory Pain
- Sex Hormone Regulation of Innate Immunity in Women and Men
- The Neural Basis of Sexually Dimorphic Brain Function
- Gender, Hormones, and Anterior Cruciate Ligament Compliance
- Regulation of Sex-Specific Genes in Drosophila

Racial/Ethnic Groups. The inclusion of different racial and ethnic groups also poses several questions. Clearly some groups remain under-represented. If the groups have been appropriately informed, why do they choose not to participate? Are the recruitment and retention strategies culturally appropriate?

Interestingly, little research has been conducted examining the rationale for participation, or lack thereof, by different racial and ethnic groups. (Ness et al. 1997) Existing studies indicate that minority groups—African-American, Native Americans, Hispanics—often do not trust White scientists, do not understand what they are being asked to do, are not recruited in a culturally-sensitive manner, and do not wish to become "guinea pigs." (Roberson 1994; Gorelick et al. 1996; Mouton et al. 1997; Stone et al. 1997; Wright et al. 1996). If, however, individuals do understand what is being asked, have an altruistic sense, and are recruited in a manner sensitive to their cultural beliefs, they are far more likely to join (Roberson 1994; Grunbaum 1996; Labarthe et al. 1996; Norton and Manson 1996; Caban 1995; Thompson et al. 1996; Whelton et al. 1996; Marquez et al. 2003; Janson, Alioto, and Boushey 2001; Royal et al. 2000; Appel et al. 1999). Given the burden of disease borne by different minority groups, increased attention is essential. Further research is imperative.

Ethical Considerations. In the rush to meet the requirements of federal funding agencies, did investigators adhere to ethical guidelines in recruiting and retaining individuals in studies? One would presume that the different institutional review boards (IRBs) necessary to submit a proposal to the NIH would be sufficient to ensure that individuals are being protected. Certainly the NIH as well as a number of IRB-related organizations have considered the issues forthrightly and diligently. Indeed, a number of conferences and educational seminars fostering and expanding understanding are held periodically across the country.

Yet, abridgement of an individual's rights is not always as clear as it seems. For example, does the promise of free medical care during trial participation, especially for an uninsured individual, affect his or her judgement? Does the promise of a substantial reward for participation entice a young man or woman in desperate need of funds? Further consideration must be given to the practice of conducting studies, presumably those that could not be ethically conducted in the United States, in other countries—especially developing nations. This issue has been raised especially in regard to AIDS trials in Africa. Is it ethical to conduct such studies in other countries even if the country's leaders and population support such studies?

Conclusions

Biomedical and behavioral investigation has advanced substantially since the beginning of the 20th century, and so have the ethical practices associated with such studies. The atrocities of the past have been acknowledged and corrective measures instituted. Where zealous regulations have occurred (exclusion of select groups of women, for example), modifications have been introduced. Individuals must now be properly informed prior to participation and cannot be coerced.

Studies now exist that examine male and female differences across racial and ethnic groups and the life span. Research funds targeting specific diseases, disorders, and conditions across the different groups continually emerge. Clinicians now have more refined data on which to base clinical interventions. More culturally sensitive resources exist for health promotion and disease prevention/intervention.

Scientific inquiry is continually challenged for even greater and more refined investigation. Issues raised by the implementation of the guidelines have in themselves provoked curiosity and questions; these questions must be addressed further. The differences between men and women must be investigated more thoroughly. Scientists and clinicians must understand what race and ethnicity contribute to health and disease. And it is imperative to understand how to embed an understanding and an appreciation for scientific inquiry and participation among all individuals. In short, the United States has come a long way, but more diversity in research is required.

References

Allen M. The dilemma for women of color in clinical trials. *J Am Med Women's Assoc*. 1994;49(4):105-109.

America's Dirty Little Secret. 2000. http://www.dc.peachnet.edu.

Appel LJ, Vollmer WM, Obarzanek E, et al. Recruitment and baseline characteristics of participants in the Dietary Approaches to Stop Hypertension trial. DASH Collaborative Research Group. *J Am Diet Assoc*. 1999;99(8 Suppl):S69-75.

Brumberg. Fasting Girls: reflections on writing the history of anorexia nervosa. *Monogr Soc Res Child Dev*. 1995;50(4-5):93-104.

Byrd WM, Clayton LA. Cancer clinical trials. Presented to the National Cancer Control Research Network Committee meeting. Boston: Harvard School of Public Health. 1992:1-13.

Caban CE. Hispanic research: Implications of the National Institutes of Health guidelines on the inclusion of women and minorities in clinical research. *J Natl Cancer Inst Monograph*. 1995;18:165-169.

Charrow RPM. Is the NIH Revitalization Act an ethnic-quota law? *J NIH Research*. 1994;6:99-101.

The Code of Federal Regulations. Title 45 CFR Part 46, Protection of Human Subjects, revised June 18, 1991.

Faden RR, TL Beauchamp. *A history and theory of informed consent*. New York: Oxford University Press; 1986.

Federal Register. Additional DHHS Protections Pertaining to Research Development, and Related Activities Involving Fetuses, Pregnant Women, and Human In Vitro Fertilization. 1998; 63(97):27797-27804.

Freedman LS, Simon MA, Foulkes, et al. Inclusion of women and minorities in clinical trials and the NIH Revitalization Act of 1993—the perspective of NIH clinical trialists. *Control Clin Trials*. 1995;16(5):277-285.

Food and Drug Administration. http://www.fda.gov/opacom/backgrounders/miles.html. 2000.

Goldstein J. *Console and Classify: The French Psychiatric Profession in the Nineteenth Century*. New York: Cambridge University Press; 1987:322-377.

Gordon. *Women's Body*. New York: Penguin; 1990:336-338.

Gorelick PB, Harris Y, Burnett B, et al. The recruitment triangle: Reasons why African Americans enroll, refuse to enroll, or voluntarily withdraw from a clinical trial. *J Natl Med Assoc*. 1998:90:141-145.

Government Accounting Office (GAO). *Women's Health: NIH Has Increased Its Efforts to Include Women in Research*. GAO/HEHS-00-96, May 2000.

Grunbaum JA, Labarthe DR, Ayars C, et al. Recruitment and enrollment for Project HeartBeat! Achieving the goals of minority inclusion. *Ethnic Dis*. 1996;6(3-4):203-212.

Hayunga E, Pinn VW. *NIH policy on the inclusion of women and minorities as subjects in clinical research*. NIH; 1999.

Janson SL, Alioto ME, Boushey HA. Asthma Clinical Trials Network. Attrition and retention of ethnically diverse subjects in a multicenter randomized controlled research trial. *Control Clin Trials*, 2001, 22(6Suppl): 236S-43S

Jones J. *Bad Blood: The Tuskegee Syphilis Experiment: A Tragedy of Race and Medicine*. New York: The Free Press; 1981.

Levine C. Women as research subjects: New priorities, new questions. In: Blank RH, Bonnicksen A, eds. *Emerging Issues In Biomedical Policy: An Annual Review*. Vol 2, New York: Columbia University Press; 1993.

Levine C. Women and HIV/AIDS. *Evaluation Review*. 1990;14(5):447-463.

Marquez MA, Muhs JM, Tosomeen A, et al. Costs and strategies in minority recruitments for osteroporosis research. *J Bone Miner Res*. 2003;18(1):3-8.

Marshall E. 1994. New law brings affirmative action to clinical research. *Science*. 1994;263:602.

McCarthy CR. Historical background of clinical trials involving women and minorities. *Academic Med*. 1994;69(9):695-698.

Meinert CL. The inclusion of women in clinical trials. *Science*. 1995;269:795-796.

Mastroianni AC, Faden R, Federman D, ed. *Women and Health Research: Ethical and Legal Issues of Including Women in Clinical Studies*. Washington, D.C.: National Academy Press; 1994.

Mouton CP, Harris S, Rovi S, et al. Barriers to Black women's participation in cancer clinical trials. *J Natl Med Assoc*. 1997;89(11):721-727.

National Academies. Committee on understanding the biology of sex and gender Differences, committee charge. Washington, D.C.: Institute of Medicine. 1999.

National Commission for the Protection of Human Subjects of Biomedical and Behavioral Research). *The Belmont Report: Ethical Principles and Guidelines for the Protection of Human Subjects of Research*. Washington, D.C.: Government Printing Office; 1978.

National Institutes of Health (NIH). NIH Workshop: Long-term effects of exposure to DES. Falls Church, Va. April 22-24, 1992. (Sponsored by the Office of Research on Women's Health and the National Institute for Environmental Health Sciences.)

National Institutes of Health Revitalization Act of 1993 (Public Law 103-43), 107 Stat 22 (codified at 42 U.S.C. § 289. a-1), June 10, 1993.

National Institutes of Health. *Outreach Notebook for the NIH Guidelines on the Inclusion of Women and Minorities as Subjects in Clinical Research*. 1994.

National Institutes of Health. *NIH Guide for Grants and Contracts*, March 18, 1994;23(11).

National Institute of Health. NIH Policy and Guidelines on the Inclusion of Children as Participants in Research Involving Human Subjects; 1998. Available at: http://www.nih.gov/guide/notice-files/not98-024.html.

National Institutes of Health. *Agenda for Research on Women's Health for the 21st Century: A Report of the Task Force on the NIH Women's Health Research Agenda for the 21st Century*. NIH Pub No. 99-4385; 1999.

National Institutes of Health. *Implementation of the NIH Guidelines on the Inclusion of Women and Minorities as Subjects in Clinical Research: Comprehensive Report (Fiscal Year 1997 Tracking Data)*; 2000a.

National Institutes of Health. NIH Computer Retrieval of Information on Scientific Projects (CRISP). Available at: http://www.nih.gov/CRISP. 2000.

Ness RB, Nelson DB, Kumanyika SK, Grisso JA. Evaluating minority recruitment into clinical studies: How good are the data? *Ann Epidemiol.* 1997;7(7):472-478.

Norton IM, Manson SM. Research in American Indian and Alaskan Native Communities: navigating the cultural universe of values and process. *J Consulting Clin Psychol.* 1996;64(5):856-860.

Piantadosi S, Wittes J. Politically correct clinical trials. *Control Clin Trials.* 1993;14:562-567.

Roberson NL. Clinical trial participation: Viewpoints from racial/ethnic groups. *Cancer Supplement.* 1994;74(9):2687-2691.

Royal C, Baffoe-Bonnie A, Kittles R, et al. Recruitment experiences in the first phase of the African American Hereditary Prostate Cancer 9AAHPC study. *Ann Epidemiol.* 2000;10(8 Suppl): S68-77.

Satel SL. Science by quota. *New Republic.* 1995:14-16.

Savitt TL. The use of Blacks for medical experimentation and demonstration in the old south. *J Southern Hist.* 1982;48:331-348.

Scull A, Favreau D. A chance to cut is a chance to cure. *Research in Law, Deviance, and Social Control.* 1986;8:3-39.

Stone VE, Mauch MY, Steger K, et al. Race, gender, drug use, and participation in AIDS clinical trials. *J Gen Intern Med.* 1997;12:150-157.

Thompson EE, Neighbors HW, Munday C, Jackson JS. Recruitment and Retention of African American patients for clinical research: An exploration of response rates in an urban psychiatric center. *J Consulting Clin Psychol.* 1996;64(5):861-867.

Tuskeegee Syphilis Study: 1932-1972. 2000. Available at: http://showme-missouri.edu/~socbrent/tusgeekee.html

Vaughn P. *The Pill on Trial.* New York: Coward-McCann. 1970;38-49.

Walker PV. NIH reports greater diversity of participants in clinical *studies. Chronicle of Higher Education.* 1996;27:A32(March 15, 1996)

Watanabe ME. 1995. NIH applicants adapt study-population inclusion guidelines. *Scientist* 1995; 9:14

Wechsler J. Micromanaging research. *Applied Clin Trials.* 1993;2:12-18.

Whelton PK, Lee JY, Kusek JW, et al. Recruitment experience in the African American Study of kidney disease and hypertension (AASK) pilot study. *Control Clin Trials.* 1996;16:17S-33S

Wittes B, Wittes J. Group therapy: research by quota. *New Republic* 1993;208(14):15-16.

Wright JT, Kusek JW, Toto RD, et al. Design and baseline characteristics of Participants in the African American study of kidney disease and hypertension (AASK) pilot study. *Control Clin Trials.* 1996;16:4S-16S.

Chapter 10

FOR-PROFIT CLINICAL TRIALS

Derrick J. Beech, MD, FACS, and
Bettina M. Beech, DrPH, MPH

Introduction

The challenge of developing new clinical therapeutics demands the interaction of the medical research industry, biomedical scientists, academic institutions, and practicing physicians. Translating data from preclinical studies into clinical practice often requires a sequence of carefully monitored trials directed toward determining the efficacy of new compounds. The impetus for creating new pharmaceutical agents and medical devices is market-driven and has intensified over the last several years as a result of the heightened understanding of disease processes. Pharmaceutical companies have strengthened their involvement in clinical trials as a component of their research and development initiatives and in response to public demands for new and more effective drugs. Direct involvement in all phases of clinical research has allowed this industry to accelerate the drug development and discovery process. Current estimates suggest that approximately 5,700 pharmaceutical agents or biotech compounds are in preclinical studies. Furthermore, an estimated 3,900 compounds are in clinical development or regulatory review (www.PhRMA.org 2003).

The introduction of genomic science has exponentially increased the number of drugs in research and development, and the costs for this research and development in the pharmaceutical industry are staggering. By the industry's own calculations, approximately 32 billion dollars was spent in 2002 on research and development by research-based pharmaceutical companies (www.PhRMA.org 2003); this figure represents a 7.7% increase in expenditures in the year 2001 and more than triple the costs from 1990 (www.PhRMA.org 2003).

The process of drug discovery begins with basic science research resulting in knowledge about disease processes, which may ultimately become the target for pharmaceutical interventions (www.PhRMA.org 2003). This information then becomes translated into the first phases of pharmaceutical product development, which is tested in clinical trials.

Clinical trials are broadly defined as studies designed to determine the efficacy of a particular therapy. Efficacy is determined by the therapeutic response, the duration of response, and survival (Held and Swedberg 1998) as they relate to the compound under investigation. Carefully conducted clinical trials provide information regarding the efficacy of a particular treatment, and they are usually the safest and fastest way for researchers (Held and Swedberg 1998) to evaluate new therapies in the clinical setting. Typically, clinical trials take place after preclinical studies have concluded that the agent or device is safe to use on humans; these earlier animal studies include dose response data as well as toxicity studies. The "gold standard" for a clinical trial is a prospective randomized clinical evaluation. These costly studies are longitudinal, well-planned evaluations and require an extensive follow-up period. Clinical trials may also assess changes in the quality and duration of life based on a particular intervention. Safety profiles with regard to toxicities and adverse events are typically included in these studies (Conti 1999).

Clinical trials are usually divided into different phases. Generally speaking, Phase I trials are primarily designed to evaluate the safety of a given treatment and the dosage needed to minimize side effects. These studies typically involve a small group of subjects and are used to detail the expected toxicities of specified therapeutic dose ranges. Phase II studies investigate new drugs or medical devices in relation to a particular disease. Phase II trials usually involve larger groups of subjects than are typically accrued in Phase I clinical trials and specifically determine the efficacy of the drug in the clinical setting. Data from Phase II trials are then used as the principal thrust for Phase III clinical studies, which typically include relatively large groups of subjects and are used to confirm the efficacy of a particular treatment. These studies usually involve the comparison of a study drug or medical device with an accepted therapy available for a particular disease. These three phases are typically considered to be the foundation for developing information to support the use of the new agent in patient care (DHHS 2000).

Phase I, II, and III studies required for Food and Drug Administration (FDA) approval account for approximately 29.1% of research and development costs for pharmaceutical companies (www.PhRMA.org 2003). Given the substantial outlay of capital in advance of a proven modality, the for-profit clinical trial industry places great emphasis on the expedient conduct of trials, particularly patient recruitment and retention.

This chapter focuses on profit-driven clinical trials and major for-profit organizations involved in clinical research. "For-profit" organizations can be broadly defined as organizations in which there is a distribution of revenues and assets to shareholders, owners, or investors. Hence, there are identifiable financial or economic gains for the organization participating in for-profit clinical research. The relevance of the involvement of these organizations in clinical trials will be evaluated in the context of the medically underserved and ethnic minority participation in these for-profit clinical studies.

The Growth of For-Profit Clinical Research

During the 1980s the majority of clinical research was conducted in academic health centers (AHC) (Lightfoot et al. 1999). Funding from government grants accounted for a large percentage of that research, holding prestige for both the medical school and the scientific investigator. At that time, seen as less prestigious than National Institutes of Health (NIH) funding, pharmaceutical companies partnered with medical schools to conduct research and produce a limited number of new products. Compensation for this research consisted of monetary payments to the university, not to individual investigators (Lightfoot et al. 1999).

Over the next 10 years, the growth of managed care changed the way in which medicine was practiced in the United States. This change included a moderation of the price of pharmaceuticals, effectively forcing the drug companies to increase the number of drugs available in the marketplace to maintain and increase their profit margins (www.PhRMA.org 2003). As a result, pharmaceutical companies increased their research and development initiatives and attempted to substantially augment their collaborations with AHCs to multiply the number of agents under investigation. However, the bureaucracies inherent in educational institutions precluded this aggressive plan of action. Academic institutions could not respond to the new pressure from drug companies to rapidly recruit participants and conduct clinical trials at the pace desired. Consequently, pharmaceutical companies began to work with private practice physicians to meet their need for speed, efficiency, and cost-effective trials (Lunik 1999; Appel 1995). Another response to this need for the consistent and efficient organization and management of clinical trials was the emergence of new research-focused companies to partner with pharmaceutical companies. Therefore, for-profit clinical trials proliferated from the pressing need for new and innovative clinical discoveries; shrinking funding for clinical research from nonprofit agencies and the NIH, and the economic and marketing incentive of industry and pharmaceutical companies to expedite newer discoveries (Appel 1995).

Key Players in For-Profit Clinical Trials

Pharmaceutical Companies

The cost of drug development in the United States is a staggering sum. Current estimates indicate that new drug discovery will cost $500–600 million dollars (Meyer et al. 1998). Not only are enormous amounts of resources spent to develop new drugs, but the length of time from discovery to market is approximately 14.2 years. Despite a provision of the FDA 1997 Modernization Act that established a "fast-track" review of drugs, the actual time from the synthesis of a new drug to its introduction into the marketplace has increased (www.PhRMA.org 2003). An increase in development time transfers into a substantial increase in the cost of new drugs; for example, a one-month delay could cost up to several million dollars (Lunik 1999).

In addition to sponsoring and financing drug trials, pharmaceutical companies are responsible for demonstrating to the FDA the safety and efficacy of investigational drugs and for the conduct of on-site monitoring of their trials. To reduce the exorbitant research and development costs and to streamline the investigational process, pharmaceutical companies began outsourcing many aspects of the conduct of clinical trials, such as the organization and management of the studies to clinical trial management groups (Lightfoot et al. 1999).

Clinical Trial Management Groups

There are a series of challenges involved in conducting clinical trials with the issue of random allocation of patients to treatment groups and statistical analysis requiring extensive resources. Data managers, research nurses, and project coordinators are needed for these clinical investigations. As a result of the stringent requirements involved in conducting prospective randomized trials, management groups and agencies have been created to assist pharmaceutical companies in data management, patient accrual, and the recruitment of study sites.

The increased requirement of large patient numbers for studies to reach statistical significance has resulted in a group of for-profit organizations that assist in the coordination of clinical trials (CenterWatch 1999). These organizations typically contract with major pharmaceutical or medical instrument companies to assist them in identifying study sites, qualifying these sites for marketing the specific research studies, and coordinating data management and specimen processing.

Clinical trial management groups (CTMGs) flourished in the late 1980s and 1990s primarily as a result of their cost-effective benefits for industries and time-efficient processing for academics. This allowed a third-party intermediary to coordinate these components of clinical research. As a result of their position, CTMGs can influence the study dynamics of a clinical trial and the validity of these studies. These intermediaries have typically been spared analysis in regard to for-profit clinical trials (Silversides 1999). However, these groups are ubiquitous in large industry-sponsored clinical research; it is rare for large-scale industry-sponsored projects to not use the assistance of a CTMG in carrying out their research objectives. Although the majority of CTMGs have no direct benefit from the actual results of studies, their involvement in these trials is a highly lucrative endeavor with significant financial rewards, regardless of study outcomes.

There are several clinical management groups, such as Clinical Investigators Pact, Ltd. (CIP), a regional trial management company that represents networks of investigators involved in clinical trials (Silversides 1999). CIP represents networks of over 3,000 investigators in the Midwest, serving a population of approximately 4,000,000 (CenterWatch 1999). This research management group has completed hundreds of studies over the last 15 years (Silversides 1999). CIP contracts with several pharmaceutical and device manufacturing companies in all phases of clinical research to help coordinate their research.

Clinical Research Organizations

Clinical research organizations (CROs) are fee-for-service, independent organizations that assist pharmaceutical companies in developing their products and bringing them to the marketplace (Lunik 1999). Many CROs have their own physicians, nurses, data managers, and laboratories, allowing the consolidation of many services (CenterWatch 1999). In addition, CROs frequently blend components of CTMGs and private and group practitioners to produce a profit-oriented organization involved in clinical trials (Woodward 2000). They are usually fiscally efficient and result-oriented, with an enormous ability to coordinate trials involving large numbers of patients in a relatively short period of time (Reed and Camargo 1999). "Clinical research organizations have evolved into a multibillion dollar industry that aids pharmaceutical firms in negotiating the labyrinth of regulatory processes" (Lunik 1999). For example, the use of CROs increased from 28% in 1993 to 60% in 1997 (Lunik 1999). The majority of this increase is due to spending on Phase II study monitoring, data management, pharmacoeconomics, analysis, and medical writing.

The nature of the relationship between pharmaceutical companies and CROs generally has two components: 1) the interpersonal component (which governs how the sponsor's project team interacts with the CRO) and 2) the corporate component (which defines the relationship between the CRO and the sponsoring company at the level of corporate interactions) (Woodward 2000). The interpersonal component is important to the degree that the pharmaceutical companies provide a supportive role to the CRO and allow their personnel to efficiently complete the contracted work. On the other hand, the corporate component is characterized by either a "one-off relationship," where the sponsor accepts bids on each project and grants the proposal to the CRO with the least expensive bid, or a "strategic relationship," where more formalized, longer-term collaborations with carefully chosen CROs are formed (Peer 1999).

Health Maintenance Organizations

The rapid growth of health maintenance organizations (HMOs) and their strict policies restricting compensation for certain clinical protocols and patients' participation in research may have contributed to the decreasing numbers of participants in clinical trials over the last several years. However, in February of 1999, the National Institutes of Health (NIH) reached an agreement with the American Association of Health Plans (AAHP), the group that oversees the managed care industry that calls for HMOs and other managed care organizations to pay for the routine costs of members who enroll in NIH-sponsored clinical trials for new drugs and medical procedures (Gifford et al. 2002). While this agreement appears to represent a considerable change in policy for HMOs, the AAHP only represents about 1,000 managed care organizations. Further, the agreement only calls for AAHP to "encourage" managed care plans to comply with the NIH plan. Managed care organizations are not required to participate; therefore, no penalties exist for maintenance of their original policies of not compensating members for experimental treatments. Lastly, the agreement only covers NIH-sponsored clinical trials. It does not include the majority of clinical trials that are sponsored by the pharmaceutical industry. Given the large number of individuals currently enrolled in some form of managed care health plan, the lack of compensation for participation can have a substantial impact on the number of potentially eligible patients who can actually access and utilize clinical health studies (Gifford et al. 2002). This is a particular consideration for ethnic minority populations, which, when insured, tend to be enrolled in an HMO, compared to a traditional fee-for-service health insurance plan. As a result, these HMOs are becoming gatekeepers for entry into clinical trials for many individuals. A recent study published in the *New England Journal of Medicine* illustrated this point regarding participation in HIV clinical trials. The researchers reported that in addition to being Black and Hispanic, that among other factors (e.g., less than a high school education and living eight miles or more from a major research hospital), belonging to an HMO reduced the likelihood of participating in a clinical trial (Gifford et al. 2002).

Clinical Academic Investigators

Pharmaceutical companies depend on clinical investigators to actually conduct clinical trials. In academic settings, clinical investigators have become increasingly burdened with coordinating the demands of the commitment to teach medical students and residents with the necessity of revenue-producing clinical productivity (CenterWatch 1999). The heralded "triple threat" of excellence in teaching, outstanding research, and expert clinical skills has become a facade in an era of diminishing federal support for academic institutions and decreasing reimbursement for clinical services (Silversides 1999). Also, academic medical institutions' dependence on clinical revenue for support of nonclinical activities further influences the academic clinician's focus on revenue-generating activities (Freeman et al. 1999). Clinical investigations do not produce revenue that directly benefits the academic investigator financially; yet these alliances allow relevant investigations that would otherwise not be performed due to limited budgets at most universities (Lind 1999). Despite the fact that clinical investigators do not benefit financially from clinical study investigations with pharmaceutical companies, other incentives are offered to these physicians, such as authorship in manuscripts. Often the pharmaceutical companies will hire "ghost writers" to write the scientific papers, but the names of successful clinical recruiters are added to the manuscripts as a "reward" (Eichenwald and Kolata 1999).

As mentioned earlier in the chapter, due to concerns about the clinical trial performance of academic health centers, pharmaceutical companies have reduced the number of clinical trials they conduct with academic clinical investigators. Because of a growing emphasis on shorter drug development times, drug companies have become concerned about the cumbersome drug-research approval process (study approval has been known to take two to five months, depending on the center); high overhead fees for clinical research; principal investigators who are overcommitted with other clinical, administrative, and teaching duties; and poor patient accrual into trials (Lunik 1999). Of further note is the higher cost of research at academic health centers compared to other sites, as well as reported higher error rates on case reports. As a result, it is estimated that academic health centers now conduct only 50% of all clinical trials in the United States (Lunik 1999), compared with 80% five years ago. Recently, however, many academic health centers are changing their infrastructure to be more responsive to the pharmaceutical industry; for example, "central support service" models have evolved that encourage communication between the investigators and sponsors, making the AHCs partners in the investigative process. Other academic medical centers have invested in infrastructure building and are forming centralized offices for clinical research. Others are working to standardize and improve quality, accessibility, and turn-around time (Lightfoot et al. 1999).

Private Practitioner Investigators

Concomitant with a decrease in the number of academic investigators conducting pharmaceutical-sponsored clinical trials has been a three-fold increase in the number of private practice physicians conducting clinical research since 1990 (Lightfoot et al. 1999). Collaboration with pharmaceutical companies has provided substantial financial benefits for these physicians. Some drug companies and their contractors offer large payments to doctors, nurses, and medical staff to recruit patients with additional incentives offered for the rapid accrual of these patients. Finder's fees are also offered for doctors who refer their own patients to other physicians who conduct clinical research (Lightfoot et al. 1999).

Pharmaceutical companies and medical device corporations frequently recruit private practitioners with high-volume practices, linking these companies with patient groups that were previously unavailable to them for medical experimentation. Private practitioners who also work as researchers, however, face several conflicts of interest. Because of the financial compensations offered, doctors are really "dual agents, with divided loyalties between the patient and the pharmaceutical companies" (Merrill 1999). Even though patients sign informed consent forms prior to joining any research study, given the delicate trust of the patient-provider relationship, patients may feel compelled to participate because their personal physician asked them to join a study. The large sum of money that can be earned by practitioners through their success in enrolling participants in clinical studies serves as an additional conflict of interest for doctors.

Clinical Trial Participants

Despite the number of variables involved in clinical trial participation, patients are the most important component in the investigative process. Without the requisite number of eligible patients, clinical studies cannot be accomplished, effectively halting the development of FDA-approved pharmaceutical interventions. Patients sought for participation in for-profit clinical trials are recruited through a variety of sources, including Internet recruitment sites, site advertisements to sponsors to recruit physician groups willing to refer patients from their practices, and newspaper advertisements from CROs.

Two provisions of the 1997 Modernization Act address the goal of appropriate representation of all population groups in clinical studies. Although the inclusion of women in clinical studies has been extensively discussed in other arenas, the issue of minority inclusion has not been equally addressed (Guy, Long, and Halperin, 1998). Even though the Modernization Act does not mandate inclusion, it does instruct the FDA to consult with NIH and pharmaceutical representatives to develop stronger guidelines regarding gender and minority parity in clinical research.

As discussed earlier, in the case of for-profit clinical trials, rapid patient enrollment is of premiere importance to the pharmaceutical companies. Without enforceable, mandatory guidelines for the inclusion of ethnic minority participants, there is little reason for the pharmaceutical industry to address this participation disparity. Substantial evidence in the literature supports many barriers to minority participation in health studies and the enormous amount of community-coordinated effort needed for successful recruitment of ethnic minority participants (Puma 1998; Cullen et al. 1994). Further, given the overrepresentation of ethnic minorities among individuals who are socially and financially disadvantaged, issues such as transportation, childcare, limited income, and homelessness often present insurmountable barriers. As reported in a recent *New England Journal of Medicine* article, most clinical trials are not designed to respond to these obstacles; therefore, study populations are rarely adequate reflections of actual treatment populations. Given these well known barriers and concerns in the enrollment of ethnic populations, coupled with the disproportionate number of uninsured members in these groups, minority populations are often omitted from health studies because they are either not asked to participate or, in many instances, do not have access to physicians who participate in clinical studies.

Ethical Controversies in For-Profit Research

The ethical issues involved in clinical trials have been extensively investigated (Gifford et al. 2002; Cullen et al. 1994; NIH Commission 1978). To ensure the ethical implementation of clinical studies, participants must not be exposed to undue harm or risk. In addition, the trial must be clinically relevant with no apparent conflicts of interests by the institutions or investigators performing the trials. Institutional Review Boards (IRBs) are the entities responsible for protecting the interests of human subjects. In 1978, the National Commission for the Protection of Human Research Subjects developed ethical principles in its' landmark document, *The Belmont Report*. The report identified important elements of informed consent, including information, comprehension, and voluntariness.

Information. Potential clinical trial participants should have clear and sufficient information that is accurate and provides a balanced perspective of the risk/benefit ratio so that an informed decision about participation can be made (DHHS 1999). Imbalanced and incorrect information may influence potential participants about joining a study. Misleading advertisements are often used to recruit participants in for-profit clinical trials. Most notable are advertisements that lead the public to believe that an investigational drug is an effective treatment, rather than an agent that is being tested in a research study (DHHS 1999).

Comprehension. A full disclosure of information about clinical studies can be overwhelming to a potential participant. Yet a clear presentation of scientific information in nontechnical language is vitally important for an informed decision regarding participation. *The Belmont Report* indicates that "presenting information in a disorganized and rapid fashion, allowing too little time for consideration or curtailing opportunities for questioning, all may adversely affect a subject's ability to make an informed choice" (McDonald 1998). Given the time pressures from drug companies to rapidly enroll participants, sufficient time is often not given to ensuring that patients fully understand informed consent documents.

Voluntariness. The last condition of the tripartite focus on informed consent is voluntariness. Despite information and comprehension of study details, risks, and benefits, decisions regarding participation must be made in an environment free from coercion and undue influence. Concerns regarding undue influences in for-profit clinical trials include large payments to participants for compensation for their time and the dual role of physician-investigators on individual decisions to participate (DHHS 1999).

Institutional Review Boards

The enormous responsibility of protecting the rights of research participants is left to Institutional Review Boards (IRBs). It is estimated that there are 3,000 to 5,000 IRBs across the country, but each functions independently of the others (Sanford 1969). IRBs that review protocols at academic health centers differ from those that review protocols for for-profit clinical trials.

University-based IRBs are predominantly comprised of physicians, professors, clergy members, and occasionally members of the lay community; most of these members serve without monetary compensation. The substantial number of protocols that must be reviewed during meetings rarely leaves time for detailed discussions and often results in incomplete review of the documents. "In some cases, the sheer number of studies necessitates that IRBs spend only one or two minutes of review per study; given time limitations, for continuing studies, these reviews may be superficially reviewed" (GAO 1996). Recent reports have documented growing concerns about the efficiency and thoroughness of the reviews and whether patients are actually receiving the safeguards against research risks that these boards are charged with protecting.

Recently, IRBs have also been formed by managed care health companies and other for-profit organizations. Although the Belmont principles are to be followed for all human subject research, for-profit IRBs are paid a predetermined fee to review protocols. Their role as a business is to review as many applications as possible, in the shortest period of time. Expediency is profitable; delays will inevitably cause clients to utilize other for-profit IRBs in the future. For example, "one federal report described the process used by some pharmaceutical companies as IRB shopping"; this means that a drug company will shop around for an IRB that will give quick approvals to proposed research protocols.

The Office for Protection from Research Risks (OPRR), a federal agency charged with the oversight of IRBs, has recently been criticized for rarely inspecting research centers. However, in response to these criticisms, this agency has become more vigilant in its monitoring of university IRBs and its record management. For example, the federally sponsored research at Duke University was temporarily shut down in May 1999 for inadequate tracking of research participants to ensure their safety. Research at the University of Illinois at Chicago was also suspended for similar lapses in human subject protocol.

Although most members of IRBs are very well intentioned and maintain high ethical standards, the sheer volume of protocols that are often required for review negates the care and attention that each protocol deserves. Some IRBs are asked to consider as many as 2,000 requests per year for the approval of drug and device studies. Other criticisms include inadequate training on the complicated ethical and scientific questions members are often faced with; little basis for knowing how well they are actually protecting human subjects; and potential conflicts of interest with industry-sponsored research (Brawley 1998).

Barriers to Minority Participation in Clinical Trials

The success of clinical trials and the ultimate success of new innovations in clinical modalities rely on the general public's receptiveness and belief that clinical investigations are safe and will ultimately contribute to the health of our society. There have been major health atrocities regarding research that have created an arena of mistrust among the general population and among minority groups in particular. Major newspapers including the *Boston Globe* led a series of front-page stories that described the treatment of several institutionalized psychiatric patients as being unethical and immoral. Additionally, the *New York Times* ran an in-depth feature on the fraudulent practices of a researcher at a major West Coast research institute (CenterWatch 1999). The newspapers' vivid account of deceptive and unethical practices along with fabricated data significantly impacts all current efforts to promote patient accrual. National magazines have also reported stories that have a negative impact on clinical trials. The May 24, 1999, editions of *USA Today* and *U.S. News and World Report* featured a story that highlighted the suspension of clinical trials at Duke University (Silversides 1998). The article repeatedly emphasized the failure of this university to appropriately respond to the federal government's Office for Protection from Research Risk. All of these issues raise serious questions about the ethical implications in clinical research and dissuade the public from actively seeking out studies in which to participate.

There has been no clinical investigation that has tainted the opinion of Americans against medical studies as much as the Tuskegee Syphilis Study (Corbie-Smith 1999). This investigation has been a strong deterrent, particularly to African-American participants, in industry-sponsored and federal investigations. The study was the longest nontherapeutic experiment on humans ever to take place in the history of medicine. Conducted and fully endorsed by the United States Public Health Services, the experiment took place between 1932 and 1972 involving 400 African-American men in Macon County, Alabama, as an observational study documenting the course of disease in these men. The unethical nature of this investigation was further heightened by the availability of effective treatments for syphilis at the origins of this investigation and then the discovery of penicillin in the 1940s, and the fact that these men were denied appropriate therapy and not counseled regarding the communicable nature of this disease and how to avoid infecting others. It was not until 1972, when the study was exposed in the mass media, that this devastating act of human exploitation was halted. Although this study ended in 1972, the effects of it continue to haunt investigators.

Minority Participation in For-Profit Clinical Trials

Involvement in clinical trials by people of color occurs in the context of continued racial bias in our society and a clear history of medical exploitation (Brawley 1998). This historic negative relationship between ethnic minorities and the research industry continues to cause challenges for inclusion of these groups.

As discussed earlier in this chapter, the growth of for-profit clinical trials has generally occurred outside of academic health centers. During the 1980s, when the majority of clinical trials were conducted in academic health centers, a large number of ethnic minority patients also received their medical care from these urban-based centers. Following the eventual decline of health studies in these settings, the access of ethnic minorities to clinical studies also declined. The move of the pharmaceutical industry into extensive collaborations with private practitioners had an effect on ethnic minority participation. Regardless of socioeconomic status, in general, the reciprocal impression of minority groups and researchers was tepid. Researchers, knowledgeable about past medical misadventures, were leery about recruiting minorities into clinical studies. Potential participants concerned about the credibility and trustworthiness of investigators were reluctant to consider research participation. These facts, coupled with the market and industry-driven pace of drug development and the need to rapidly recruit a large number of participants, effectively removed ethnic minority participants from participating in for-profit clinical studies in significant numbers. Although some NIH clinical trials have achieved a proportionate number of minority participants, these trials have been the exception, rather than the rule. Further, the cost associated with the intensive strategies needed to accomplish this goal can be significant, and beyond either the monetary or time scope of most studies.

Conclusion

The continued underrepresentation of minority participants in health studies poses significant problems for reducing health disparities in the United States. "The bioethical principle of social justice requires that a fair share of the burdens and benefits associated with participating in research be distributed within a society" (Corbie-Smith 1999). Risks associated with research participation should not be understated; however, the societal benefits of the outcomes of studies tend to far outweigh the potential drawbacks. As scientific discoveries occur on a daily basis, the result of limited participation on the part of groups of color indicates that scientists will have incomplete knowledge of the effectiveness of new modalities on all groups. Although science has not demonstrated a reason for racial and ethnic variation in drug efficacy or metabolism, the degree of generalizability of research findings from any homogenous group cannot scientifically and comfortably be extrapolated to a heterogenous population. Therefore, committed efforts to be as inclusive as possible in for-profit clinical trials will further ensure that all groups will equally share the benefits of bio-medical and behavioral interventions to improve population health.

References

Appel A. Advisors may urge NIH to seek out industry support for clinical trails. *Nature*. 1995; 378:116.

Brawley OW. The Study of Untreated Syphilis in the Negro Male. *Int J Radiation Oncology Biol Phys*. 1998;40(1):5-8.

CenterWatch, 6(6): June 1999. Copyright 1999.

Corbie-Smith G. The Continuing Legacy of the Tuskegee Syphilis Study: Considerations for Clinical Investigation. *Am J Med Sci*. 1999:317(1):5-8.

Conti CR. Clinical Trials and the cost of Medical Care. *Clin Cardiol*. 1999;22:549-550.

Cullen MR, Upton A, Buffler P, Robins T, Schenker M, Fine L, Wiencek R, Widess E, Chiazze L. The private funding of public research. *J Occup Med*. 1994;36(12):1348-1354.

Department of Health and Human Services (DHHS). *Recruiting subjects: Pressures in Industry-Sponsored Clinical Research*. Office of Inspector General, 2000:OEI-01-97-00195.

Eichenwald K, Kolata G. A doctor's drug trials turn into fraud. *New York Times*, 1999, May 17.

Freeman WR, Bartsch D, Mueller AJ, Banker AS. Innovation and Clinical Trials. *Arch Ophthalmol*. 1999;117:846-847.

Gifford AL. Participation in research and access to experimental treatments by HIV-infected patients. *N Engl J Med*. 2002;346(18):1373-82.

Gorelick, PB, Harris Y, Burnett B, Bonecutter FJ. The recruitment triangle: Reasons why African-Americans enroll, refuse to enroll, or voluntarily withdraw from a clinical trial. *J Natl Med Assoc*. 1998;90:141-145.

Guy G, Long P, Halperin J. Minority Accrual to Clinical Trials—Minority recruitment strategies for the breast cancer prevention trial. *Oncology Iss*. 1998;13(4):26-27.

Held P, Swedberg K. To Screen or Not to Screen: How to improve clinical trials. *J Cardiac Failure*. 1998;4(3):237-238.

Lightfoot G, Getz K, Harwood F, Hovde M, Rauscher S, Reilly P, Voger J. Faster time to market: ACRP's white paper on future trends. *Appl Clin Trials*. 1999;April;56-68.

Lind S. Financial issues and incentives related to clinical research and innovative therapies. In: Vanderpool. *The Ethics of Research*. 1999;185-202.

Lunik M. Clinical research: Managing the issues. *Am J Health Syst Pharm*. 1999;56:170-174.

McDonald J. Clinical tests on humans called flawed; trials for new drugs, medical devices said to expose subjects to unnecessary risks. *Hartford Courant*, 1998: June 12.

Merrill R. Modernizing the FDA: An incremental revolution. *Health Affairs*. Mar-April 1999.

Meyer M, Genel M, Altman RD, Williams MA, Allen JR. *Clinical Research: Assessing the Future in a Changing Environment; Summary Report of Conference Sponsored by the American Medical Association Council on Scientific Affairs*, Washington, D.C., March 1996. Am J Med 1998; 104:264-271.

The NIH Commission for the Protection for Human Subjects and Biomedical and Behavioral Research. *The Belmont report: Ethical principles for the protection of human subjects of research*. Washington, D.C.: U.S. Government Printing Office, 1978.

Peer R. Managed-care plans agree to help pay the costs of their members in clinical trials. *New York Times*. February 9, 1999.

Puma JL. Researching for-profit research: the obligations of hospital ethicists. *Clin Res*. 1998:569-73.

Reed CR, Camargo CA. Recent Trends and Controversies in Industry-sponsored Clinical Trials. *Academic Emerg Med*. 1999;6(8):833-839.

Ruffmann R. Funding of Clinical Research. *Lancet*. 1999;354(14):602.

Sanford JP. Has Clinical Research Failed in Its Public Trust? *Clin Res*. 1969;XVII(3):577-580.

Silversides A. Private sector becoming the key to research funding in Canada. *CMAJ*. 1998;159:397-8.

Woodward R. Keys to developing an effective outsourcing strategies. *BioPharm*. 2000;13(2):22-26.

www.PhRMA.org/publications/publications/profile02.index.cfm. Accessed September 1, 2003.

Zapol NJ. Negotiating industry-sponsored clinical trial agreements: a view from the trenches. *Ann N Y Acad Sci*. 2001:949:349-51.

Chapter 11

ACADEMIC HEALTH CENTERS and COMPETITIVE FORCES in HEALTH CARE:
Implications for Research on Problems of the Underserved

David Blumenthal, MD, PhD, Eric G. Campbell, PhD, and Joel S. Weissman, PhD

Introduction

Much has been written about the effects of financial stress on academic health centers (AHCs) and their missions (research, education, care of vulnerable populations, provision of rare and highly specialized services) (Commonwealth Fund Task Force on Academic Health Centers 1997, 1999a, 2002, 2001; Levin, Moy, and Griner 2000; Moy et al. 1997; Moy et al. 2000). This work has repeatedly made the point that AHCs have historically used clinical surpluses to cross-subsidize their mission-related activities, but that those surpluses, which accumulated generously prior to the early 1990s, have been less abundant since that time. During the period from 1994 to 1998, the primary reason for these declining margins was the price pressures exerted by managed care organizations (MCOs) on providers in a number of local markets around the United States. Since 1998, another factor has come into play: the implementation of the Balanced Budget Act of 1997, which reduced payments to all hospitals under Medicare Part A, graduate medical education payments to teaching hospitals in particular, disproportionate-share payments to hospitals, and payments to home health care organizations. Unlike competitive forces, which vary markedly from market to market around the U.S., the Balanced Budget Amendment of 1997 (BBA) has exerted a more uniform effect on AHC margins country-wide (Weissman and MacDonald 2000).

From the standpoint of public policy, the financial fortunes of AHCs have importance primarily to the extent that they affect valued social activities. AHCs play a unique or disproportionate role in producing a number of goods and services that are generally accepted as important to the health and welfare of our citizens. Though these activities are rarely unique to academic health centers, AHCs often make unique contributions to these missions. In the case of research, AHCs perform much of the basic health science research in the U.S. and play a predominant role in translational clinical research, through which basic research findings are first applied to the problems of patients (Commonwealth Fund Task Force on Academic Health Centers 1999b; Association of American Medical Colleges 2000a). In education, AHCs are almost uniquely responsible for the undergraduate medical education of health professionals and train approximately half of all postgraduate physicians, including the overwhelming majority of future academic physicians, the next generation of teachers and researchers (Commonwealth Fund Task Force on Academic Health Centers 2000). In the clinical arena, AHCs provide disproportionate amounts of highly specialized and high technology services and disproportionate amounts of service to low-income populations (Commonwealth Fund Task Force on Academic Health Centers 1999b).

The Commonwealth Task Force on Academic Health Centers has been studying whether the evolution of market pressures in health care has affected any of these contributions to social welfare, also known as social or public goods. Some of the salient findings are briefly summarized below. In addition, in this chapter we address an important and under-investigated aspect of this issue, that is, whether financial pressures on AHCs may disproportionately and adversely affect vulnerable populations, and most particularly, whether research on the problems of these populations may be at risk.

There is some reason to single out research—and especially clinical research—on the problems of the underserved as vulnerable under current circumstances. AHCs are uniquely positioned to conduct research on the health problems that disproportionately affect low-income patients and underrepresented minorities These problems include HIV/AIDs, tuberculosis, sexually transmitted diseases, substance abuse, homelessness and its associated health problems, domestic violence, child abuse, premature and low birth weight deliveries, malnutrition, and, increasingly, the rare (in the U.S) infectious illnesses that burgeoning immigrant populations are bringing to North America (Commonwealth Fund Task Force on Academic Health Centers 1999b). Low-income citizens and underrepresented minorities also disproportionately encounter a series of social and economic problems that can adversely affect their health: barriers to access to services, racial discrimination, lack of insurance, and poverty in general. AHCs tend to be physically located in the inner city areas, where patients with these problems are concentrated. Physical proximity makes it easier for researchers at these institutions to design and execute studies that take into account not only the biological but also the critical social and environmental influences on the conditions in question. The fact that vulnerable populations tend to utilize AHCs—and especially publicly owned AHCs—more commonly than other institutions creates the necessary critical mass of patients to make clinical research feasible.

Unfortunately, few data exist on the amounts of research conducted by AHCs (or other institutions) on the problems of low-income patients and underrepresented minorities, nor is much known directly about how these types of investigations have fared over the last five years. This chapter, therefore, can be seen as a conceptual exploration of this topic, generating hypotheses for future investigations.

That exploration proceeds in the following manner. First we review the evidence that AHCs are facing increased financial pressures, and that these pressures threaten their ability to cross-subsidize their missions. Second, we review the special role of AHCs in caring for the indigent, and how that role may be evolving under the pressure of the competitive marketplace. Third, we discuss what is known about the research missions of AHCs, and how these in particular, including research on poor and indigent patients, may be affected by the changing circumstances of AHCs. In a fourth section, we review some responses of AHCs to the pressures of the health care marketplace, and how these responses themselves may affect research on the indigent. A brief concluding section closes the chapter.

Added Costs of AHC Missions

In the U.S. health care system, several forces have converged to make it difficult for hospitals to increase or even maintain current levels of payment for their services. The growth in managed care and competitive forces generally have resulted in a widespread belief in prudent purchasing among virtually all health plans and payers. The passage of the BBA portends lower payments from Medicare. The nation's teaching hospitals may be especially impacted by these changes in the marketplace because they are more costly than community hospitals.

The nation's 125 AHCs educate a variety of individuals, including medical students, residents, graduate students, and postdoctoral fellows in the life sciences as well as students in the allied health sciences. Because involving trainees in clinical activities is not conducive to efficient practice, these activities result in higher costs of treating patients. Furthermore, most persons familiar with AHCs understand that education of students and medical residents is just one factor that contributes to higher costs of patient care. Inefficiencies or cost add-ons in support of performing clinical research, or resources devoted to maintaining stand-by capabilities for essential community services like burn units and trauma centers, also contribute to the higher costs of patient care. In the past, the magnitude of these costs have been difficult to estimate.

In its initial report, "Leveling the Playing Field," the Commonwealth Fund Task Force on Academic Health Centers estimated the total cost of graduate medical education (GME) and other mission-related activities in 1997 to be $18.1 billion based on an all-payer econometric model from the Lewin Group (Commonwealth Fund Task Force on Academic Health Centers 1997). This estimate was consistent with others based directly on Medicare program payments. Using January 1997 baseline estimates from the Congressional Budget Office (CBO), Medicare paid an estimated $7.1 billion for GME. Extrapolating these figures to all patients based on the share of business represented by Medicare patients results in an estimate in 1997 that ranges from $16.5 billion to $20.3 billion. The Lewin estimate fell just below the midpoint of this range. This analysis was updated subsequently by Lewin Associates, and the cost of GME and other related activities in 2002 was estimated to be $27.2 billion. In a separate analysis, the Lewin Group estimated the effects on costs due to the provision of specialty services, stand-by capacity for specialized programs such as burn care, and clinical research. The findings from the regression models were used to decompose costs per case into four elements: base costs, case-mix, labor-related variables (wages and staffing), and mission-related costs. The mission-related costs can then be further subdivided into three components: GME, stand-by capacity, and clinical research. The result of this calculation, by level of teaching activity for 1999, is shown in Figure 1, which confirms the relationship between these groups of variables and the added costs of academic health centers.

Until recently, the higher costs of teaching hospitals have been paid either by explicit subsidies from state governments or by charging insured patients more, a practice known as cost-shifting. In some regions of the country, teaching hospitals have been able to continue extracting higher payments from private patients due to their reputation for higher quality. However, the ability of AHCs to cost-shift is at risk under competitive forms of health care, and may no longer be tenable. As demonstrated by Figure 2, the ratio of payments to costs for private payers has been declining since the early 1990s. Chief financial officers of teaching hospitals understand that these declining rates mean that it will be more and more difficult to expect commercial payers, including HMOs, to pay the added costs necessary to support AHC missions.

Besides cross-subsidies from private payers, for the past 20 years teaching hospitals also have collected special payments from Medicare to cover the higher costs of patient care due to academic missions. However, academic health centers also are beginning to see decreases in teaching payments from Medicare as a result of provisions in the Balanced Budget Amendment of 1997. Although the decreases were

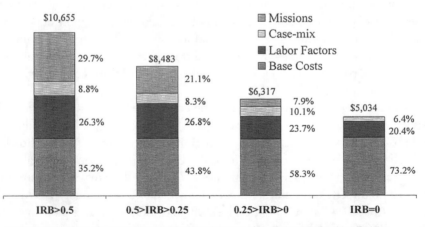

Source: Georgetown University analysis of data in Coleman et.al., Estimating Provider, Training, Standby Capacity and Clinical Research Costs Using Regression Analysis. Lewin Associates, 1999

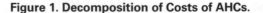

Figure 1. Decomposition of Costs of AHCs.

mitigated to some extent in the Balanced Budget Refinement Act of 1999 and the Medicare, Medicaid, and SCHIP Benefits Improvement and Protection Act of 2000, the total reduction to American hospitals generally is still expected to be more than $100 billion from 1998 to 2004 (Levin, Moy, and Griner 2000).

These changes in the marketplace and public policy have had a noticeable impact on the finances of several of the nation's premier academic health centers—the flag-ship hospitals that have the largest commitment to teaching and research. Their financial fortunes have taken a decided downturn. While the majority are finan-cially solvent, AHCs' average margins were at historic lows, declining from 5.3 to 2.6 percent between 1996 and 1999 (Association of American Medical Colleges 2000a). Furthermore, the major teaching hospitals at 14 of the 18 most research intensive AHCs experienced 1999 operating losses, down-grades of their credit sta-tus, or negative outlooks from one of the major bond rating agencies. In addition, some well known institutions—the University of Pennsylvania, the Beth-Israel Deaconess Medical Center in Boston, Georgetown University Medical Center, University of Minnesota, Detroit Medical Center, University of California San Francisco—have had severe losses requiring dramatic countermeasures, including the sales of university hospitals or large-scale layoffs. For the first time in history, an academic health system (Allegheny Health Education and Research Foundation) went bankrupt in 1999.

Although many institutions, especially in less competitive markets, continue to have healthy bottom lines, there is no way to know with certainty whether the nation's AHCs as a group will emerge stronger or weaker from current stresses, or how their social missions will be affected in the process. Given the vanishing mar-gins of teaching hospitals, it is likely that cross subsidies for education, research, and patient care activities have declined or, in some instances, disappeared (Association of American Medical Colleges 2000b). As put by the chairman of a clinical depart-ment in one of the nations most competitive health care markets, "It is difficult to

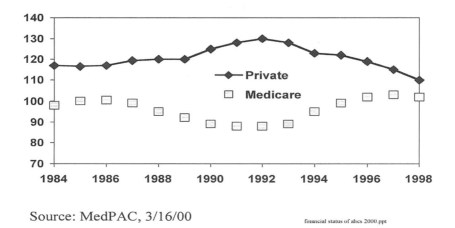

Source: MedPAC, 3/16/00   financial status of ahcs 2000.ppt

Figure 2. Payment-to-Cost Ratios for Private Payers and Medicare.

use revenues to continue to subsidize the research and education missions of the department when you are asking faculty members to go without raises or even take pay cuts." As a result of the changes that some AHCs are experiencing, some observers worry that AHCs overall may be faced with reductions in the productivity and competitiveness of their research enterprises, in the quality of educational experiences for undergraduate and graduate health professionals, and in their ability to sustain current levels of care to indigent patients.

The Indigent Care Mission of AHCs

Research, education, and care to the poor have long been intertwined in the American medical education establishment, and have their roots in the development of the hospital, itself. The primary concern of early hospitals was not with medical care, per se, but with philanthropic and spiritual goals. These institutions offered solace and shelter to lepers, orphans, invalids, and travelers. The habit of AHCs to care for disadvantaged patients grew out of these philanthropic traditions. Yet with the advent of modern medicine and its evolution as a costly component of our nation's economy, hospitals went "… from treating the poor for the sake of charity to treating the rich for the sake of revenue" (Starr 1982). Charity care became, to some extent, the cost of doing business in the community.

As medical care becomes more commercialized, there is growing concern that the emphasis on the bottom line is making the tradition of indigent care less tenable, which has clear implications for researchers on problems of low-income and minority patients. In the same way that Willie Sutton preferred to rob banks due to the presence of money in their vaults, clinical researchers interested in problems of disadvantaged persons prefer access to indigent patients in their everyday practice in order to understand the problems of this population, and to facilitate their enrollment in clinical protocols. Despite their roots as charitable institutions, the evidence on the role of teaching hospitals in caring for low-income, minority, and disadvantaged patients is mixed. Some studies have shown little association between teaching status and indigent care, while others demonstrate substantial service to underserved patients that is growing fastest in very competitive markets.

The provision of indigent care has been the subject of investigation by the Prospective Payment Assessment Commission (ProPAC), the agency that reports to Congress on Medicare policy. This issue has been controversial, because Medicare's Indirect Medical Education (IME) adjustment for teaching hospitals is seen by some as a way to offset some of the costs of indigent care. The results of this research have not supported the idea of a strong association between teaching and indigent care, at least with respect to uncompensated care.* After netting out public subsidies meant to offset the direct costs of indigent care, ProPAC found little statistical rela-

---

* Uncompensated care is normally defined as the sum of free care and bad debts. Together they account for approximately 6% of hospital costs. Free care alone accounts for about 1–1.5% of total costs, although in practice it is difficult to separate true charity from bad debt due to hospitals' discretion in implementing collection policies. The level of uncompensated care is related to the number of uninsured persons and the number of persons with inadequate private insurance (Weissman 1996).

tionship between the size of a hospital's teaching program and the level of uncompensated care it provides (Ashby 1991; Ashby 1992; Prospective Payment Assessment Commission 1995).

However, uncompensated care is only one measure of a hospital's commitment to caring for disadvantaged patients. Since the beginning of the program in 1965, Medicaid patients have turned to teaching hospitals to receive the care they needed. Serving large numbers of Medicaid beneficiaries often signals hospitals' interest in welcoming vulnerable patients. ProPAC analyses have shown that major public teaching hospitals attributed nearly a third of their patient care costs to Medicaid services. The figure for major private teaching hospitals was 16%, but only 11% and 10% for minor teaching and nonteaching hospitals (Ashby and Harris 1995). Although some hospitals that treat a disproportionate number of indigent patients are able to obtain enough public payments to meet or even exceed their costs, many other teaching hospitals lose substantial sums of money on their Medicaid cases.

Other studies have taken into account both uncompensated care and care to Medicaid patients as a measure of a hospital's commitment to serving the poor. One of the earliest studies of care to the poor by teaching hospitals in the Medicaid era used the sum of Medicaid charges, charity (for patients who are deemed unable to pay after meeting certain criteria), and bad debt (for patients who presumably can afford to pay, but don't). Members of the Council on Teaching Hospitals (COTH) were considered to be major teaching hospitals. In 1980, private COTH hospitals accounted for 22% of indigent care by this definition, yet comprised only 15% of all hospital beds; likewise, public COTH hospitals provided 16% of care to the poor, yet only represented 5% of all hospital beds. More than a decade later, researchers at the AAMC employed a similar approach to measure indigent care at teaching hospitals, referring instead to number of patients served rather than encumbered charges (Association of American Medical Colleges 1998). Looking at the proportion of patients who were classified as self-pay, charity, or insured by Medicaid, the gap between teaching hospitals and other hospitals that persisted throughout the time period (Figure 3) narrowed a bit during the mid-1990s, but teaching hospitals still provided more care to indigent patients than did other hospitals as of 1995.

One reason for the high level of indigent care provided by AHCs is that many are state-owned institutions. Public support is often provided with the understanding that these facilities function as providers of last resort. Researchers at Georgetown have found that teaching hospitals provide more charity care regardless of ownership status. AHCs and other major teaching hospitals provide higher levels of charity care as a percentage of their gross patient revenue than other hospitals in the same ownership category (Figure 4). The same study showed that AHCs account for a disproportionate share of indigent care in their communities—28% of uninsured admissions versus about a 16% share of all admissions.

Whatever the past experience of AHCs with indigent care, the future may be less certain. On the one hand, the higher costs of academic health centers discourage price-sensitive purchasers from sending patients to their facilities. For example, an analysis by the Task Force in 1996 showed that AHCs receive less than their expect-

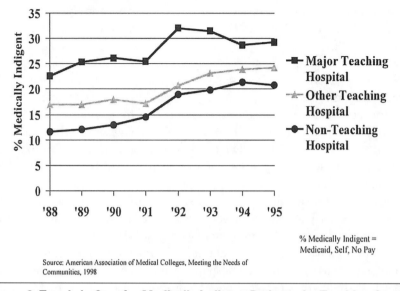

Source: American Association of Medical Colleges, Meeting the Needs of Communities, 1998

Figure 3. Trends in Care for Medically Indigent Patients, by Teaching Status, 1988–1995.

ed share of managed care patients (Commonwealth Fund Task Force on Academic Health Centers 1997, 2001). Medicaid managed care seems to have the same effect in some instances. In a study of Tennessee's TennCare program, it was found that Medicaid patients in managed care plans sometimes switched their care to lower cost community hospitals (Meyer and Blumenthal 1996). In particular, it was reported that the routine, and often more profitable, obstetric patients and their babies tended to be admitted to community hospitals, leaving the high-risk, complex, and costly patients to the public teaching hospital.

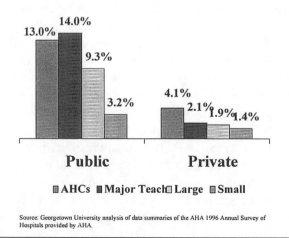

Source: Georgetown University analysis of data summaries of the AHA 1996 Annual Survey of Hospitals provided by AHA.

Figure 4. Charity Care as a Percentage of Gross Patient Revenues, 1996.

On the other hand, one expected outcome of competition in health care markets is that certain hospitals will exhibit a diminishing willingness to care for uninsured patients, leaving the responsibility to others. Due to their reputation as safety net institutions, AHCs have begun to experience an increase in the proportion of patients unable to pay for their care. In 1991, AHCs accounted for about 40% of the charity care provided in their communities, with private AHCs responsible for 11% and public AHCs for about 30%. Five years later, this figure increased to 44%, with private and public AHCs' shares totaling about 13.5% and 30.7%, respectively (Figure 5). The move toward greater competition has not occurred evenly across all areas of the U.S. As a result, the trend toward greater concentration of indigent care has varied, depending on the competitiveness of the local market. After classifying MSAs according to the penetration rate of managed care, there was little, if any, increase in indigent care concentration between 1991 and 1996 in less competitive markets. Most of the increase in AHCs' market share of indigent services occurred in highly competitive markets.

While most attention has been placed on patients at financial risk, another way to think about vulnerable patients is to consider groups that, by virtue of their social, demographic, economic, or clinical status, are at risk for being underserved. Racial minorities, for example, or patients with diseases that are difficult to treat, often have difficulties accessing the medical care establishment, and major teaching hospitals have done their share in treating these patients. The AAMC examined the distribution of patients who met three categories of medical vulnerability—medically indigent (Medicaid or uninsured), low income, and minority (Black or Latino). Patients with multiple risk factors were considered to be at heightened risk of experiencing barriers to timely and high quality medical care. The proportion of these multiple-risk patients at major teaching hospitals was twice that of minor teaching hospitals and four times the number admitted to nonteaching hospitals. Similarly, in 1996, about 26% of all inpatient AIDS cases were admitted to AHCs, which accounted

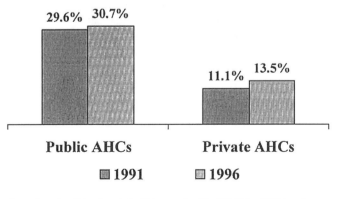

Source: Georgetown University analysis of data summaries of the AHA 1991 and 1996 Annual Surveys of Hospitals provided by AHA.

Figure 5. Share of Total Charity Care Provided in Communities, 1991 and 1996.

for just 6% of hospitals and 13% of beds in the communities studied (Georgetown analysis). Also revealing, the share of AIDS cases varied dramatically by insurance status. AHCs provided care for 36% of all hospitalized AIDS patients insured by Medicaid, 34% of uninsured cases, but only 15% of privately insured and 3% of HMO AIDS cases (Georgetown).

The ability of teaching hospitals to continue serving all patients regardless of ability to pay is under increasing pressure as health markets become more price conscious. Whether they can actually increase this role, without sacrificing other missions or their economic survival, remains to be seen. In the short term, there are structural reasons why AHCs will probably continue to treat high proportions of the nation's neediest individuals. AHCs are most often found in core urban centers, where the demand for indigent care is most concentrated. Only three (University of West Virginia, Dartmouth, and Iowa) are located outside of a metropolitan area. Furthermore, nearly half (44%) of AHCs are publicly owned facilities (Reuter and Gaskin 1998). In the short term, therefore, the fear that patients traditionally seen in AHCs (specifically people of color) are being removed in large numbers from sites where clinical trials are being conducted seems to be unfounded. In the long term, the stresses associated with providing care to poor and uninsured patients could, in the current price-conscious health care market, reduce the ability of AHCs to continue their traditional role as safety net institutions and their ability to conduct research on the problems of indigent patients.

Research

The importance of internal clinical cross-subsidies for the support of AHC missions is as well demonstrated for research as for any other AHC mission. Most observers agree that for every dollar in external research support received, AHCs must contribute between 15 and 20 cents of internal funds (Commonwealth Fund Task Force on Academic Health Centers 1999; Snyderman 1998). It is therefore reasonable to hypothesize that financial competition among local institutions for patient volumes would reduce the surpluses necessary to cross-subsidize research, and potentially reduce the efficacy of AHC research investments. Evidence from a variety of sources tends to confirm this hypothesis. First, a 1994 study of the behavior and attitudes in research-intensive AHCs demonstrated that clinical faculty in highly competitive markets reported lower rates of publication in peer-reviewed journals than did peers in less competitive markets (Campbell et al. 1997). Faculty in competitive markets also reported higher rates of conflict and lower rates of cooperation within their departments than did faculty in more tranquil locales. Second, studies in the mid-1990s by the Association of American Medical Colleges demonstrated that rates of growth in NIH funding tended to be lower among AHCs in markets with high degrees of managed care penetration compared to AHCs in areas where managed care was less active (Moy et al. 2000). Third, data on internal subsidies provided by AHCs to support the work of their investigators showed that AHCs in highly competitive markets tended to be less generous to their investigators than did AHCs in less competitive locales (Weissman et al. 1999).

An unanswered question is whether reductions in federal Medicare payments may intensify the forces that have produced these effects on the research missions of AHCs. It may take some years before the consequences of these changes in federal policy are apparent, one way or another, and they will almost certainly be masked to some extent by increases in NIH funding for the direct costs of research. The latter increases, in fact, could conceivably make reductions in available internal cross-subsidies largely irrelevant. While this rosy scenario is not implausible, there remains reason for concern. First, the requirement for institutions to match NIH funding with internal monies has not gone away; thus, massive increases in NIH funding could have the perverse effect of placing even greater strain on the ability of AHCs to maintain their full range of missions. One interesting indicator of stress induced by Medicare cuts, competition, and increasing NIH funding would be whether AHCs actually decide to decline some NIH funds because of lack of internal matching support.

The proliferation of managed care and competitive models of health care have affected the way clinical trials are performed in AHCs. Reflecting intense pressure from employers to contain costs of care, MCOs are hesitant to sanction enrollment of patients in some clinical trials because of the extra clinical costs associated with experimental treatments or experimental protocols. The Commonwealth Fund Task Force on Academic Health Centers has investigated these matters and found that many clinical investigators believe that managed care organizations discourage enrollment in clinical trials. This occurs via a variety of mechanisms. Some managed care plans simply do not allow patients to participate in clinical trials, while in other cases enrollment is difficult and requires the direct intervention of the PI. Some plans will not pay for complications associated with new investigational protocols if the patients are randomized to the experimental arm(s) of the study. Other managed care companies have been reported to discourage patient enrollment in clinical trials by taking too long to make decisions about patient participation or by reimbursing at levels sufficiently low to discourage physician participation.

One of the most consistently mentioned barriers to enrolling patients in trials is that physicians practicing in today's competitive environments no longer have the time to attend to activities other than patient care. The pressures on physicians to be more clinically productive in highly competitive markets tend to reduce the time they have to recruit patients into trials, a process that often extends visits to explain the rationale for the experiment and to provide informed consent. Simply put, money and time are the biggest barriers to enrolling patients, including the time spent getting informed consent, and documenting the care patients receive.

Finally, reductions in federal Medicare payments may disproportionately affect research on the problems of underserved patients. For reasons already noted, AHCs with large burdens of indigent care are best positioned to conduct research on the problems of the underserved. This is particularly true for AHCs whose major clinical facilities are municipal or county hospitals, where indigent patients tend to congregate for their care. These facilities have few privately insured patients, and their clinical incomes are thus heavily dependent on Medicare and Medicaid payments, and on such extra payments as graduate medical education and disproportionate share reimbursements under Medicare. Both graduate medical education and disproportionate share payments were significantly reduced under provisions of the BBA, and so-called refinements of the BBA have not restored those payments to previous levels.

Responses of Academic Health Centers to Financial Pressures

Academic health centers have responded to the changing health care environment with a number of internal changes that could have implications for research on the problems of the poor, uninsured, and underrepresented minorities. Among these changes, the most pertinent may be the decisions of some AHCs to distance themselves from their clinical missions and the decisions of others to invest large portions of their reserves in the development of community-based primary care networks.

The first of these responses, a reduced involvement in provision of clinical services, is apparent in AHC sales of teaching hospitals and sometimes faculty group practices to nonacademic hospital chains. Among the AHCs who have taken this step are Georgetown Medical Center in Washington, D.C., Tulane University Medical Center in New Orleans, Washington University Medical Center in Washington, D.C., University of Minnesota Medical Center in Minneapolis–St. Paul, and Creighton University in Omaha, Nebraska. In other cases, such as the University of North Carolina at Chapel Hill, state authorities have reduced involvement of the academic institution in the governance of its clinical affiliates, splitting off the clinical operation into a separately managed, state-owned entity.

The motivations for these maneuvers vary. Some are intended to reduce the exposure of the AHC and its parent university to financial losses on the part of the clinical enterprise, while others are simply intended to improve the management of clinical facilities. Whatever the intent, the general strategy may have the effect of distancing researchers from clinicians, and reducing the commitment of clinical administrators to the research missions of their academic partners. To the extent that the facilities in question serve indigent patients and have been or could be important sites for clinical investigation on the problems of the poor and underrepresented, the consequences could be the erection of additional barriers to research on the problems of this patient population. Among the institutions mentioned above, at least two have played major roles in caring for indigent patients in their communities: George Washington University and Creighton University. Neither of these institutions, however, has had major research commitments of any kind. More recently, there have been discussions of increasing the independence of the health systems of the University of Pennsylvania and Duke University from their parent universities. The former, in particular, has a major commitment to the underserved in Philadelphia. The long-term consequences of such potential reforms in AHC governance need careful monitoring for all of their missions, including effects, if any, on research on underserved populations.

A second response on the part of AHCs to financial pressures, and particularly, to the advent of managed care, has been the development of regional networks of primary care physicians owned by or affiliated with the academic health center. This strategy has proven to be a major financial drain on some of the institutions that have undertaken it, in part because several, such as the University of Pennsylvania, expended large sums in purchasing primary care practices, often at inflated rates. Even institutions that avoided this pitfall, such as Partners HealthCare System in Boston, nevertheless face substantial expenditures to create the information systems and other infrastructure required to integrate these community practices into a single health care enterprise.

The development of community-based primary care networks has potential benefits and pitfalls for research on the problems of the underserved. On the one hand, the investment of scarce capital in the creation of these systems reduces surpluses available to cross-subsidize research of all kinds, including research on the underserved. Investments in development of primary care networks has played a role in generating substantial operating losses at the University of Pennsylvania, the University of San Diego Medical Center, and Beth Israel–Deaconness Medical Center in Boston.

On the other hand, some of the new networks created by AHCs feature community-based facilities, including community health centers, that serve substantial numbers of poor and underrepresented minorities. This has been true, for example, in the cases of Partners HealthCare System (which strengthened its ties with several community health centers as part of its network development), Vanderbilt Medical Center (which developed a partnership with nearby Meharry Medical College as part of its response to the TennCare program), and the University of San Diego Medical Center (which developed relationships with several primary care practices serving Medicaid populations in the mid-1990s). The creation of new roots in underserved communities creates access to indigent populations that were not previously available to faculty at these AHCs. Whether the motivation and resources to further utilize this opportunity will materialize remains to be seen.

Summary and Conclusion

In the current turmoil of the health care system, the activities of academic health centers face challenges. Since neither AHCs nor the organizations that monitor them collect systematic data on the health or robustness of AHC missions, finding definitive evidence on the status of these missions is difficult. This is particularly true of selected mission-related activities, such as research on the problems of poor and underserved populations.

Nevertheless, the indirect evidence from a number of sources presented in this chapter suggests that research on problems of the poor and underserved shares the vulnerability of AHC missions generally. AHCs are suffering from financial stresses to their clinical operations, resulting in unprecedented declines in operating margins. These margins have been critical to subsidizing research in the past. Because they treat disproportionate numbers of indigent patients, AHCs are uniquely positioned to investigate the problems of these patients. Thus, there is every reason to suspect that the general threat to research activities will affect research on the problems of this population.

What this will mean for the health care of the poor and underserved over the long term is difficult to say with certainty. During the late 1990s, the U.S. enjoyed a brief reprieve from the relentlessly increasing numbers of uninsured in our population (EBRI 2001). The principal causes of the lower numbers were a strong economy with more workers in higher wage jobs, flat growth in premiums, and expansion of the State Children's Health Insurance Program, which decreased the number of uninsured poor children. However, these encouraging trends are likely to be only temporary. Furthermore, there is other evidence that increased competition in health care results in greater concentration of indigent care among fewer providers, especially among AHCs (Commonwealth Fund Task Force on Academic Health Centers 2001). At a time of rising insurance premiums and drug costs, the likelihood that the health system will expand coverage for the poor is extremely remote. What this means for the future role of AHCs in caring for poor and vulnerable members of society remains to be seen.

References

Ashby J. *The Trend and Distribution of Hospital Uncompensated Care Costs, 1980-1989*. Washington, D.C.: ProPAC; 1991.

Ashby JL, Jr. The burden of uncompensated care grows. *Healthc Financ Manage*. 1992;46(4):66, 68, 70–2 passim.

Ashby J, Harris J. *Hospital Costs and Payments by Revenue Source: The Impact of Medicaid Payment Increases in 1992*. Washington, D.C.: Prospective Payment Assessment Commission; 1995.

Association of American Medical Colleges. *AAMC Data Book 2000*. Washington, D.C.: AAMC; 2000a.

Association of American Medical Colleges. *AAMC Fact Sheet: The Financial Health of Teaching Hospitals Continues to Decline*. Washington, D.C.: AAMC; 2000b.

Association of American Medical Colleges. *Breaking the Scientific Bottleneck in Clinical Research: A National Call to Action*. Washington, D.C.: AAMC; 2000c.

Association of American Medical Colleges. *Meeting the needs of communities: How medical schools and teaching hospitals ensure access to clinical services*. Washington, D.C.: AAMC; 1998.

Campbell EG, Weissman JS, Blumenthal D. Relationship between market competition and the activities and attitudes of medical school faculty. *JAMA*. 1997;278(3):222–6.

Commonwealth Fund Task Force On Academic Health Centers. *A Shared Responsibility: AHCs and the Provision of Care to the Poor and Uninsured*. Washington, D.C.: The Commonwealth Fund; 2001.

Commonwealth Fund Task Force on Academic Health Centers. *From Bench to Bedside: Preserving the Research Mission of Academic Health Centers*. Washington, D.C.: Commonwealth Fund; 1999a.

Commonwealth Fund Task Force on Academic Health Centers. *Leveling the Playing Field: Financing the Missions of Academic Health Centers*. New York: The Commonwealth Fund; 1997.

Commonwealth Fund Task Force on Academic Health Centers. *Patterns of Specialty Care: Academic Health Centers and the Patient Care Mission*. Washington, D.C.: Commonwealth Fund; 1999b.

Commonwealth Fund Task Force On Academic Health Centers. *Training Tomorrow's Doctors: The Medical Education Mission of AHCs*. Washington, D.C.: The Commonwealth Fund; 2002.

Commonwealth Fund Task Force on Academic Health Centers. Unpublished Analyses of 1996 Medicare Data by E. Valente. Washington, D.C.: AAMC; 2000.

EBRI. *Sources of Health Insurance*. Washington, D.C.: 2001.

Levin R, Moy E, Griner PF. Trends in specialized surgical procedures at teaching and nonteaching hospitals. *Health Aff* (Millwood). 2000;19(1):230–8.

Meyer GS, Blumenthal D. TennCare and academic medical centers: the lessons from Tennessee [see comments]. *JAMA*. 1996;276(9):672–6.

Moy E, et al. Distribution of research awards from the National Institutes of Health among medical schools. *N Engl J Med.* 2000;342(4):250–5.

Moy E, et al. Relationship between National Institutes of Health research awards to US medical schools and managed care market penetration. *JAMA.* 1997;278(3):217–21.

Prospective Payment Assessment Commission. *Medicare and the American Health Care System: Report to Congress.* Washington, D.C.: Prospective Payment Assessment Commission (ProPAC); 1995.

Reuter J, Gaskin G. The Role of Academic Health Centers and Teaching Hospitals in Providing Care for the Poor. In: Altman SH, Reinhardt UE, Shields AE, eds. *The future U.S. healthcare system: who will care for the poor and uninsured?* Chicago: Health Administration Press; 1998.

Snyderman R. Restructuring the Research Enterprise for the Future. In: Rubin E, ed. *Mission Management: A New Synthesis.* Washington, D.C.: Association of Academic Health Centers. 1998;2:408.

Starr P. *The social transformation of American medicine.* New York: Basic Books; 1982.

Weissman J. Uncompensated hospital care. Will it be there if we need it? *JAMA.* 1996;276(10): 823–8.

Weissman J, MacDonald E. *Current Findings on the Financial Status of Academic Health Centers.* Cincinnati: Commonwealth Fund Task Force on Academic Health Centers; 2000.

Weissman JS, et al. Market forces and unsponsored research in academic health centers. *JAMA.* 1999;281(12):1093–8.

Chapter 12

COMPLEMENTARY AND ALTERNATIVE MEDICINE:
A Challenge for Health Researchers

Maurine Goodman, MA, MPH,
Joe Jacobs, MD, MPH,
and Bettina M. Beech, DrPH, MPH

Introduction

Complementary and alternative medicine (CAM), as defined in the medical literature, consists of systems and practices for treating disease and promoting health which are not an integral part of conventional medicine and practices, not taught in most medical schools as therapies to be used on patients, and not offered as therapies in most U.S. hospitals (Crock et al. 2000; NCCAM 2001). If these systems and practices are used as therapies in addition to allopathic medical therapy (biomedicine), they are complementary. If they are used instead of allopathic medicine, they are alternative. CAM therapies, reasons for CAM use, and utilization patterns all vary substantially by culture, ethnicity, and socioeconomic status. Kaptchuk and Eisenberg refer to CAM users as "a heterogeneous population promoting disparate beliefs and practices that vary considerably from one movement or tradition to another and form no consistent body of knowledge" (Kaptchuk and Eisenberg 2000).

The use of CAM therapies to prevent and treat illness is a fundamental aspect of health behavior that all patients have in common (Hufford 1997). Complementary and alternative medicine includes such diverse therapies as chicken soup for colds, herbal medicine, faith healing, acupuncture, therapeutic massage, megavitamins, macrobiotics and other nutritional therapies, self-help groups, energy healing, homeopathy, hypnosis, quigong, yoga, and therapeutic touch. It includes Mexican-American Curanderismo, Native American medicine, Espiritismo, traditional Chinese medicine, Indian Ayurvedic medicine, and humoral medicine (hot-cold theory). Some form of CAM is utilized by people in all sectors of society from the least to most educated, from poorest to richest. It is practiced by individuals on themselves and their families or obtained through practitioners. A primary feature of CAM is its cultural foundation. All human systems for maintaining health, preventing illness, and healing sickness are deeply rooted in a set of beliefs and values that are cultural in nature. And "nothing, it seems, is as difficult for human beings as to have their belief systems challenged" (Jobst 1999).

CAM use among participants in health studies presents several problems for investigators. Of primary concern is that CAM utilization may interfere with treatment that is part of the research study, affect study outcomes, hinder compliance, and hinder continued participation. Underlying these problems is the cross-cultural gap between people who are allopathic medical professionals and people who are not. When the researcher and participant are of different racial, ethnic, or socioeconomic backgrounds, the cultural distance is even wider, making it more difficult to establish the high level of trust that is essential for open communication about the participant's health beliefs and practices (Pachter 1994). Study participants may use CAM without the researcher's knowledge and without knowing the importance of disclosure. And while the actual CAM therapies may affect study outcomes, so can the patient's health beliefs affect treatment response. These are some of the reasons that health researchers should be aware of CAM use by members of their target population, acknowledge it, and be able to communicate about it to patients—perhaps accepting it as complementary treatment if not harmful.

Many forms of CAM that are deeply rooted in the cultural traditions of particular ethnic groups now appeal to a much broader group of consumers. Once considered solely as the prescientific healing traditions of the poor and uneducated, CAM is now a multibillion dollar industry in the United States. The following section gives an overview of this highly visible and highly commercial aspect of CAM, which is sweeping the country and propelling CAM into the realm of the allopathic medical profession and industry. The remaining sections of the chapter provide a conceptual framework for understanding complementary and alternative medicine as part of a culturally based health care system that pertains to all people, regardless of race, ethnicity, or socioeconomic background, while highlighting practices that are of importance in minority communities. Finally, we will offer suggestions for a culturally competent approach for discovering and discussing the health beliefs and practices of research participants.

The Rising Acceptance of CAM

Consumers

In 1980, when Arthur Kleinman wrote *Patients and Healers in the Context of Culture*, he observed "a recrudescence of traditional healing" in contemporary western society. As much now as it did then, the phenomenon creates a difficult question for medical professionals and society in general, "what to do about folk practitioners in planning for health care" (Kleinman 1980). Folk practices (another term for CAM) are not fading away; they are becoming more prevalent as new forms emerge to suit the sensibilities of Americans not entirely satisfied with allopathic medicine as their only source of health care.

The explosion of interest in CAM within the medical community has been driven in large part by the increasing use of CAM therapies among well-educated, middle-class Americans (Jobst 1999). This highly visible, highly articulated category of CAM, which has received a tremendous amount of media coverage, both print and electronic, is the one most familiar to Americans. It includes a wide range of practices and therapies including relaxation therapy; massage; herbal therapies; homeopathy; aromatherapy; chiropractic; self-help; energy healing through magnets, Therapeutic Touch, and Reiki; nutritional therapies such as megavitamins, macrobiotics, and other special diets; yoga and other exercise therapies; acupuncture (Eisenberg et al. 1998). It also includes various " 'New Age' revisions of practices from other cultures" such as Navajo medicine and Chinese traditional medicine (Hufford 1997). Numerous volumes describing and prescribing these modern CAM therapies line the health-section shelves of mega-bookstores, and those therapies that can be packaged fill the shelves of large, modern drug stores. And the World Wide Web is a major source of communication for this very "cosmopolitan" version of complementary and alternative medicine (Hufford 1997).

Several studies focusing on various cosmopolitan CAM therapies have offered profiles of its users (Berman et al. 1998; Eisenberg et al. 1998; Owens, Taylor, and Degood 1999). One frequently cited study that surveyed the use of 16 popular CAM therapies reports that CAM use is most common in the West among college-educated people with incomes greater than $50,000, more common among women, and less common among Blacks (Eisenberg et al. 1998). Others have characterized this level of CAM user as a "cultural creative," part of an emerging group of individuals who are open to new experience, think holistically, and place high values on art and aesthetic experience. They were found to have a positive affect and strong sense of well being (Owens, Taylor, and Degood 1999). Stephen Straus, director of the National Center for Complementary and Alternative Medicine (NCCAM), goes right to the point, stating that "CAM enjoys particular popularity among baby boomers" (Straus 2000).

While traditional medical practices are thought by many to pass down from one generation to the next, cosmopolitan CAM users are as likely to learn these health behaviors from books, magazines, mail order catalogs, and the Internet. As stated previously, large bookstore chains have devoted major sections to CAM literature, and there is evidence that an abundance of CAM users are connected to the World Wide Web. In early 2000, the NCCAM reported that its website was averaging 460,000 hits per month (Straus 2000). Nonetheless, cosmopolitan CAM is every bit a cultural phenomenon as the more traditional practices that thrive in minority communities, but that are less visible to nonminority groups.

So why do educated western consumers, acquainted with the effectiveness of modern allopathic medicine, turn away to try new therapies yet to be evaluated in clinical trials? Many reasons have been offered. High on the list is a holistic view of health: a philosophical orientation that emphasizes the importance of mind, body, and spirit and treatments that focus on the "whole individual." Preferring treatments that they perceive as more humane and less likely to cause harm, they are attracted to therapies that address the nutritional, emotional, and lifestyle factors affecting health (Astin et al. 2000; Berman et al. 1998; Millet 1999). Kaptchuk and Eisenberg suggest that the "persuasive and compelling nature" of CAM may have less to do with effectiveness and more with its cultural premises, which include an advocacy of nature, vitalism, "science," and spirituality. These aspects of CAM offer patients "a participatory experience of empowerment, authenticity, and enlarged self-identity when illness threatens their sense of intactness and connection to the world." By adopting natural treatments and changing one's lifestyle to a more "natural" existence, one becomes a more authentic and less artificial person. There is a preference for the vitalistic forces of therapies such as Tai Chi, Ayurvedic medicine, and homeopathy, which are seen as more natural and life-enhancing than drugs and surgery, which are seen as artificial and destructive of life. Also driving use of cosmopolitan CAM therapies is a growing belief in the form of vitalism that emphasizes a mind-body connection and healing through imagination, will, and belief (Kaptchuk and Eisenberg 2000).

These reasons for CAM use are popularly associated with "New Age"" thinking, a strongly middle-class phenomenon in the United States. According to Hopwood, "New Age" thought arose among well-educated middle-class persons who felt somewhat alienated from their own culture and ambivalent about the increasing influence of science and materialism. A feature of New Age thinking is "a strong attraction to practically all folk belief traditions which are seen to possess a spirituality [which] antedates the corrupting influences of modern materialism" (Hopwood 1997). And while most cosmopolitan CAM consists of revised versions of ancient healing traditions, there are many healing beliefs and practices popular in minority communities that are not a part of cosmopolitan CAM.

The characteristics of cosmopolitan CAM and its users, including their reasons for use, contrast strongly with CAM therapies and practices in minority populations in the U.S. Among the many differences, perhaps the one most responsible for the widespread and growing acceptance of CAM in the biomedical community is the high socioeconomic status of cosmopolitan users. College-educated and wealthy, they are closer to the academic culture of biomedicine and its practitioners than are minorities of lower socioeconomic status. They have greater access to care; they have greater spending power; and they receive more respect and attention from the biomedical community than most minorities in the United States, especially those who are less educated, have lower incomes, and speak English as a second language. Although the majority of cosmopolitan CAM users do not discuss their nonconventional practices with their physicians; their preferences are shown by their spending, and their demand is driving the supply (Eisenberg et al. 1998; Pachter et al. 1998; Wynia, Eisenberg, and Wilson 1999).

The Biomedical Profession and Industry

The widespread and increasing consumer demand for complementary and alternative therapies has given rise to increased awareness and acceptance of CAM within the biomedical community. While some sectors embrace CAM as a growth market with potentially large financial gains, others are more concerned with the safety of patients who use CAM therapies that are potentially harmful or incompatible with biomedical therapies (Berman et al. 1998; Bhattacharya 2000; Devries 1999; Eskinazi and Muehsam 2000; Jobst 1999; Kaptchuk and Eisenberg 2000; NCCAM 2001; Pachter 1994). In most cases, the interest and concern has been directed toward cosmopolitan CAM therapies and the people who use them (Hufford 1997; Pachter 1994).

Strong consumer demand for CAM has been documented by Eisenberg et al. who found that 42% of U.S. healthcare consumers spent a total of $27 billion on out-of-pocket expenditures for alternative medicine in 1997 compared to $29.3 billion spent for all U.S. physician services that same year (Eisenberg et al. 1998). Recognizing that CAM is "big business, HMOs, hospitals, and primary care groups have begun offering CAM therapies to their clients" (Jobst 1999). The pharmaceutical industry has also responded to consumer demand by marketing herbal remedies once available only in health food stores. In 2000, the industry estimated the therapeutic herbal market at $3 billion, a figure expected to grow to $25 billion in less than a decade. In light of the potential financial gains, the industry has offered to support trials to evaluate the efficacy of botanicals purchased as complementary and alternative therapies (Eskinazi and Muehsam 2000). It is likely that these figures are the "tip of the iceberg" since they concentrate on one category of CAM within one major socioeconomic group; nonetheless, they are increasingly presented in the literature as a defining feature of CAM.

The change in biomedicine is also indicated by an increasing number of training programs that offer courses about CAM, and health professionals who accept CAM to some degree. Citing a study published in 1998, the NCCAM reports that 75 out of 117 U.S. medical schools offered elective courses in CAM or included CAM topics in required courses (NCCAM 2001). Medical schools also offer continuing education programs on CAM for practicing physicians (Bhattacharya 2000; Devries 1999). Parallel to the growth in CAM training is greater acceptance of CAM by physicians. Several studies have demonstrated that a growing number of physicians accept CAM, refer their patients for CAM treatment, use CAM treatment themselves, and receive training in actual CAM practices (Astin et al. 2000; Berman et al. 1998; Crock et al. 2000; Pachter et al. 1998; Wynia, Eisenberg, and Wilson 1999). Astin et al. report that large numbers of physicians are either referring patients for CAM therapies or practicing "some of the more prominent and well-known forms of CAM" (Astin et al. 2000). In a study of CAM attitudes and practice patterns among primary care physicians, Berman and colleagues found increasing usage of CAM practices that "until recently have been unheard of or shunned by the medical establishment." Their study, which focused on 19 popular CAM therapies, also revealed that many physicians have been trained in CAM and use it, with younger physicians expressing the most positive attitudes toward CAM practices. Highest on the list of CAM therapies accepted and practiced by physicians are the mind-body therapies of biofeedback and relaxation, counseling and psychotherapy, behavioral medicine, and diet and exercise. Chiropractic and acupuncture are also highly accepted by physicians in the U.S. According to Berman et al., these therapies conform "to the structural definition of complementary and alternative medicine . . . not generally taught in U.S. medical school and institutions," and they serve as examples "of therapies that have moved with time from the fringe to the mainstream" (Berman et al. 1998). There has also been increased acceptance among other health professionals; for example, "tens of thousands" of nurses have been trained in Therapeutic Touch, a form of energy healing, and use it in clinical practice (Eskinazi and Muehsam 2000). Again, cosmopolitan CAM is the category of greatest acceptance and familiarity in biomedicine.

Medical Research and Government

Interest in CAM extends to the medical research community and the U.S. government through its National Center for Complementary and Alternative Medicine. Established in 1992 as an office within the National Institutes of Health, NCCAM's primary objective is to disseminate information about the safety and effectiveness of CAM practices. The NCCAM supports basic and clinical research and research training on CAM, and it provides information about CAM to health care providers and the public. Its budget grew from $2 million in 1993 to $68.7 million in 2000 (NCCAM 2001).

To date, most research supported by NCCAM has focused on cosmopolitan therapies; but its focus is expanding to include research in minority populations. In its "Strategic Plan to Address Racial and Ethnic Disparities," NCCAM acknowledges a lack of information on, reasons for, variations in, and outcomes of CAM use in minority populations, and that this information is needed for effectively addressing excess morbidity and death in racial and ethnic minority populations. As part of this initiative, NCCAM has committed research funds for "identifying and understanding the gaps in knowledge regarding CAM use in minority populations." The expanded program will include studies on safety and effectiveness, but also qualitative research to understand health behaviors and the meaning of therapeutic practices within the context of particular cultures (NCCAM 2001).

It is good that the NCCAM is broadening its research agenda to include studies on CAM in minority populations; the information generated through this extremely important initiative will certainly be helpful to physicians and health researchers who work with minority patients. But we are not at ground zero in understanding minority use of CAM; therefore, the new NCCAM research will build upon a strong foundation of knowledge already laid by anthropologists, sociologists, and physicians as a result of their vast experience with healing practices among minorities groups, including Native Americans; African-Americans; populations originating in different areas of Latin America, Southeast Asia, and Europe; and other groups who are minorities in the United States. Much of this ongoing research is published in social science journals, and much of it predates the biomedical community's interest in CAM. As CAM research continues in both fields, the NCCAM will provide a much needed infrastructure for sharing information about CAM across disciplines and with the public.

Although social scientists and medical researchers have focused their studies on different categories of CAM use, there is strong agreement that CAM is a cultural phenomenon—part of a complex, culturally based health care system that governs what people believe about health and what they do to maintain it. It is more than a set of remedies for illnesses favored by particular groups of people; CAM includes beliefs, attitudes, and observations about what causes illness and how it should be prevented or healed (Hufford 1996). Psychiatrist and anthropologist Arthur Kleinman has developed a model of health care systems that all disciplines can use as a framework for understanding human healing practices in all cultures, including one's own. The following section introduces the major components of this model as a framework for discussing minority CAM practices in relation to those of the majority population and conventional biomedicine.

Kleinman's model helps us to move beyond racial and ethnic classifications of CAM, emphasizing its applicability to all groups and its importance in health care. Although most CAM therapies utilized in the United States originated within racial and ethnic populations, in practice, one cannot assume a particular minority patient knows about or uses any of the CAM therapies associated with his or her group. In communicating with patients about their health beliefs and practices, it is important to maintain awareness that significant CAM practices may be used while avoiding stereotypes that associate individual patients with specific practices. Finally, the health care systems model emphasizes the cultural significance of CAM for all groups.

Health, Culture, and CAM: Kleinman's Model

Health Care Systems

When thinking about "health care systems" most people in the United States focus on the biomedical system of care, which includes hospitals, physician practices, pharmaceuticals, public health activities, etc. However, in the larger context of human healing behavior, this biomedical system of care is one of many ways of dealing with illness. In the United States, it is part of a larger cultural system that includes beliefs about the causes of illness, norms governing the choice and evaluation of treatment, status and power relationships, and interaction settings and institutions (Kleinman 1980).

In Kleinman's model, health care systems are organized through the interaction of many variables, including interpersonal relationships (e.g., doctor–patient, patient–family, social network), interaction settings (e.g., home, doctor's office), social institutions (e.g., clinics, hospitals, professional associations, health bureaucracies), economic and political constraints, available treatment options, and others. All health care systems consist of three overlapping sectors: popular, folk, and professional, and health maintenance (prevention), recognition of illness (diagnosis), and treatment occur in all three. Each sector can be seen as a separate subculture with different values, beliefs, practices, ways of communicating, and rules of behavior. Allopathic medicine (scientific biomedicine) fits within the professional sector of this framework (Kleinman 1980). Complementary and alternative medicine fits within all three. This model accommodates all categories of CAM practices and can be used "across cultural, historical, and social boundaries [to] explain the inner workings of clinical care: illness behavior, practitioner–patient transactions, and healing mechanisms." The sectors connect as patients move from one to another as they make decisions about their health (Kleinman 1980).

The Popular Sector (Self-Care)

The popular sector of every health care system is the "lay, nonprofessional, non-specialist, popular culture arena" where illness is first recognized and acted upon, where patients decide what to do about their illness and whether to treat it themselves without the assistance of a practitioner. It is within this sector that patients evaluate treatment plans they've received from practitioners and decide whether to comply, whether the treatment was effective, and whether they are satisfied with its quality. The popular sector is comprised of a matrix containing several levels: individual, family, social network, and community beliefs and activities (Kleinman 1980). It is an important part of the health care system of all human populations. Health researchers should be familiar with popular sector practices for the following reasons.

Popular sector care is prevalent and varied in research populations. Within the category of indigenous healing traditions, popular sector practices (self, family, and community-based care) are the most active and widely used part of every health care system (Kleinman 1980). Between 70% and 90% of all illness episodes are managed within the popular sector via self or family care, before consulting any type of practitioner, and it is common for these therapies to be used in addition to those prescribed by biomedical clinicians. Most health behavior within this sector is oriented toward maintaining health and preventing illness rather than treating sickness (Kleinman 1980).

Popular sector healing practices are based on what people believe is good for themselves and their families. They include whatever people do to maintain good health or treat an illness. Ranging from practices familiar to physicians to exotic traditions studied by anthropologists, they include dietary requirements and restrictions, herbalism, sanitation practices, exercise, avoidance of certain substances, over-the-counter remedies, and spiritualism; some examples are chicken soup for colds, teas for stomach problems and everything else, cranberry juice for urinary tract infections, yogurt for stomach ailments, and garlic for heart health or keeping away worms or evil spirits. They include widely varying practices for keeping one's self, family, and home "clean," wearing of amulets or specific colors, bleeding, sweating, burning, cutting, vomiting, etc.

While some practices from this sector are benign, others might interfere with biomedical research outcomes by affecting symptoms and/or the action of medications being studied. For example, common Puerto Rican folk therapies for treating childhood asthma involve harmless practices such as "praying to the saints," assisted by use of a prayer candle and other forms of spiritism such as wearing Azabache, a Black stone, to protect one from evil influences (Pachter, Cloutier, and Bernstein 1995). Other potentially harmful practices include the use of elemental mercury in spirit cleansing ceremonies; syrups that include concentrations of witch hazel that could produce toxic effects if ingested in sufficient amounts; and rubs that include higher than recommended concentrations of camphor (Pachter, Cloutier, and Bernstein 1995). (Pachter et al. provide specific recommendations for reacting to these and other folk therapies in clinical practice.) Others have reported therapies that involve ingesting lead-containing substances (Risser 1995).

Popular sector therapies may be used by more than one group. When discussing differences between categories of CAM, minority practices are commonly referred to as ethnomedicine or folk medicine, while cosmopolitan practices are simply referred to as CAM (Hufford 1997; Pachter et al. 1998; Pachter 1994). But from the standpoint of biomedicine, all popular sector practices are complementary and alternative (to biomedicine). Ethnomedicine or folk medicine may be correctly seen as a category or subset of CAM, which differs from cosmopolitan CAM in many ways; however, many therapies are common to both, although utilized with different frequency. For example, a study by Pachter et al. demonstrated that European and ethnic minority families use home-based practices for treating illness with similar frequency, even after controlling for economic and demographic differences. The major differences were in the relative frequency of specific remedies and in categories of CAM. In their survey of European-Americans, African-Americans, Puerto Ricans, and West Indian-Caribbeans, all groups reported use of camphor rubs such as Vick's Vapo Rub for treating colds. However Puerto Ricans utilized this therapy more frequently than the Europeans and African-Americans. And counter to conventional wisdom among CAM researchers, the practice of humoral medicine (hot-cold theory) for treating colds was found to be practiced more frequently by European Americans than African-Americans, Puerto Ricans, and West Indian- Caribbean respondents (Pachter et al. 1998). (Hot-cold theory refers to traditional practices used to treat and prevent illness by achieving balance or homeostasis by combining foods, diseases, and practices that are culturally identified as having "hot" or "cold" qualities. The quality of "hot" or "cold" in hot-cold therapies does not necessarily refer to temperature; and what is considered "hot" or "cold" varies by culture for the same foods, remedies, and practices.)

Such cross-cultural surveys assist health researchers in understanding patterns of CAM use by minorities. Knowledge of therapies used and the frequency of use within in a study population is an important starting point for effective communication with patients. However, it is of greater importance to know that popular sector, home-based therapies constitute the most common form of health care among all groups, and that many factors, such as health, education, religious affiliation, ethnicity, occupation, and social network, influence how patients perceive and use health resources within the health care system (Kleinman 1980). It is neither a "New Age" nor an ethnic phenomenon, and researchers can never assume that a particular patient uses a particular type of CAM therapy, regardless of ethnicity or socioeconomic background.

Most patients don't disclose CAM. Most patients do not initiate discussions about home remedies with biomedical providers, especially if they perceive cultural distance or expect to meet with disapproval (Eisenberg et al. 1998; Pachter et al. 1998; Pachter 1994; Wynia, Eisenberg, and Wilson 1999). Cultural distance between practitioners and patients may result from differences in education and financial and social status; language differences; and differences in how each understands health and illness. It affects the quality of clinician-client interactions, and is more likely in studies involving racial and ethnic minorities (Pachter 1994). With cultural distance, there is a greater chance for miscommunication resulting in distrust and an unwillingness to join a study or continue in one. When it is important to know about a patient's health beliefs and practices, it is essential to approach the topic in a respectful and nonjudgmental way (Flores 2000; Hopwood 1997; Hufford 1996; Pachter 1994).

The Folk Sector (Folk Practitioners)

The folk sector, a part of all health systems, is closely related to the popular sector. It is the domain of the nonprofessional, nonbureaucratic specialists who people consult about health problems. In Kleinman's classification, folk practitioners are those who are not organized into professional societies. They generally lack uniform guidelines, training, literature, certification, and licensure. Their craft is acquired through generational transfer and apprenticeships rather than through an organized profession. Folk practitioners are considered by their clients to have specialized knowledge and abilities about healing.

Some other distinctive features of folk medicine are that:

- It is heavily dependent on oral transmission (*although influenced by print and occasionally producing booklets, tracts, and other publications*);

- It is relatively informal in structure (*although specialists may be trained through formal apprenticeship*); and

- It is relatively noncommercial (*although folk specialists (e.g., traditional herbalists) may receive some cash payments or barter*) (Hufford 1997).

Healing practices by folk practitioners include sacred and secular healing, "herbalism, traditional surgical and manipulative treatments, special systems of exercise, and symbolic, nonsacred healing" (Kleinman 1980). Some examples include shamans, psychics, voodoo priestesses, cuaranderas, etc. Navajo healing traditions include several types of healers—"diagnosticians such as hand tremblers, crystal gazers, and listeners, to individuals who perform healing ceremonies involving herbs, balms, and purgatives" (Kim and Kwok 1998).

A primary difference between the folk and popular sectors is that the healing practice is performed by someone outside the family environment. It is not self-care. In some less developed societies lacking professionalization, the entire health care system is dominated by the folk and popular sectors (Kleinman 1980).

The decision to consult a folk healer is rooted in beliefs and values of the popular culture. It has little to do with whether biomedicine is available or dominant within the larger health care system. Patients often perceive folk healers as the most accessible specialists for health care assistance due to shared values, culture, and language. Studies have shown that use of traditional healers in addition to biomedicine is common in ethnic populations, and that this folk practice is not commonly discussed with biomedical practitioners (Flores 2000; Kim and Kwok 1998; Pachter et al. 1998).

Wherever there are ethnic populations with different ideas about healing, there are folk practitioners available to help. Even when folk healers are expensive and inconvenient (distance, long waiting times), people use them for healing. In virtually every community with large ethnic populations, one can find folk healers with thriving practices and long waiting lists. This is of particular concern for researchers striving to recruit minorities with cultural orientations and healing traditions that do not regard biomedicine as dominant.

The Professional Sector (Organized Healing Professions)

In Kleinman's model, the professional sector consists of all organized healing professions, which he refers to as professional subsectors. Modern scientific medicine falls within this category. Also included are professionalized indigenous medical systems such as Chinese traditional medicine and Indian Ayurvedic medicine (Kleinman 1980). Unlike folk medicine, professional sector medicine is characterized by some level of institutionalization with practice guidelines, special training, licensure, certifications, literature, and legitimacy within the societies where they exist. In the United States, the professional subsectors, including CAM therapies, rely increasingly on communication technology media, so that its practices are rapidly transmitted to many different regions and many sectors of society. This results in similar practices within each professional subsector, including CAM, wherever they are found (Hufford 1997).

An important characteristic of the professional sector is each group's struggle for dominance within the health care system. In the competition for dominance or legitimacy, we have seen healing practices, once in the folk sector, become organized and move into the professional sector. For example, acupuncture, once regarded as a fringe, folk medical practice in the United States, is now widely researched, sought after by patients, and practiced by licensed specialists including MDs with dual training (Astin et al. 2000; Berman et al. 1998). The same can be said of herbal medicine, which is rapidly moving into the realm of established pharmaceutical companies along with increasing interest and concern by United States government agencies. A majority of the CAM modalities practiced in this country have arisen from the traditional healing practices of other nations.

In the history of western medicine, it took a long time for biomedicine to achieve dominance, finally becoming equated with the very definition of medicine (Millet 1999). As other healing practices make "their claim for place and acknowledgment as legitimate practices, they become understood as alternatives to the dominance of biomedicine." Within the health care system model, and from the perspective of patients who use CAM, biomedicine is itself an alternative—dominant, but one method among others that are available and trusted.

Implications for Research Practice

Health researchers should be aware that traditional healing practices thrive in racial and ethnic communities and that these culturally based health systems are very stable and resistant to change (Hufford 1997). Minorities who favor traditional health practices may be the least willing to abandon their beliefs about what healing methods work, to participate in a study that falls within the framework of conventional medicine. If they perceive insensitivity to their beliefs and cultural distance between themselves and researchers, their reluctance may be reinforced to the point of alienation. And finally, what patients believe about illness and health frequently affects treatment outcomes, an association being investigated in many studies of CAM therapies.

For ethnic minorities who choose to participate in health studies, chances are high that they won't initiate a discussion about their CAM beliefs and practices with researchers. Studies show that approximately 70% of CAM users do not tell their physicians about their CAM practices, and most biomedical practitioners are uncomfortable discussing the topic for various reasons (Crock et al. 2000; Pachter 1994). It is reasonable to assume that this communication problem within the clinical setting holds true in research practice. If so, the researcher is left in the dark about CAM practices that might affect study outcomes by influencing a patient's decision to join a study, comply with treatment protocols, or continue participation.

Just as clinical practice among diverse populations can be enhanced by a culturally competent approach to patient beliefs and practices, so can research practice. When interviewing participants to find out about their health beliefs and practices, consider the following guidelines:

1. Initiate discussions with research participants about their beliefs and practices in a sensitive and nonjudgmental manner.

2. Remember that CAM practices vary widely within racial and ethnic minority populations. Patients who identify with a racial or ethnic minority do not necessarily subscribe to particular health beliefs or practices associated with that group. For example, a Mexican American woman who has never and would never consult a curandera (folk healer) might take offense at any assumption or implication that she would.

3. Remember that the terms "complementary and alternative medicine," "folk medicine," "ethnomedicine," "cosmopolitan medicine," and "folk healers" are used by health professionals and social scientists to describe health practices. People do not use these terms to refer to their own health practices and may be offended or too embarrassed to respond.

4. Avoiding the term "beliefs and practices," ask the participant to share what he or she knows about the health condition associated with the research project and whether other family members or friends have had the condition. This is one way to find out about patient beliefs. What family members and friends think and do about a health condition may provide clues about the patient's own health beliefs and practices.

5. To discover practices that involve folk or professional healers, ask whether the participant (or participant's family member or friend) has received any kind of treatment for the health problem. If so, ask the patient to describe the treatment, the amount of treatment if applicable, and the frequency. Ask whether

the treatment helped at all—whether the patient felt better. (It is not important at this point whether the researcher thinks the treatment is effective. The point is to find out what the patient believes!)

6. To discover popular sector (self-treatment) practices, ask whether the participant (or family member or friend) has tried anything to prevent or treat the health problem. If so, ask him or her to describe the treatment.

7. If the patient begins to discuss what he or she thinks is the cause of the problem, listen carefully! Remember that beliefs about cause give rise to remedies.

8. If the patient has engaged in or may participate in alternative treatments, determine whether they are harmful or will have an effect on study outcomes. If the alternative treatment has the potential for serious harm, it must be discouraged, but in a sensitive and respectful way (Pachter 1994).

9. If the alternative treatment is not harmful, do not attempt to dissuade the patient from his or her beliefs, but educate him or her about the biomedical therapy that is part of the research project and the importance of complying with research protocols. Combining alternative and biomedical therapies may help increase compliance since doing so places the biomedical therapy "within the context of the patient's cultural system and lifestyle" (Pachter 1994).

The most important issue for researchers regarding CAM is the cross-cultural gap between people who are biomedical professionals and people who are not. Bridging that gap requires more than knowledge of particular CAM therapies associated with specific racial and ethnic groups. It requires open, respectful, and nonjudgmental communication, initiated by the clinician, in order to establish trust and appropriate compliance with study requirements.

References

Astin JA, Marie A, Pelletier K, Hansen E, Haskell WL. A review of the incorporation of complementary and alternative medicine by mainstream physicians [Review Article]. *Arch Intern Med* [serial online]. 1998;158(21):2303-2310. Available from: Ovid Technologies, Inc. Accessed April 23, 2000.

Astin JA. Why patients use alternative medicine: results of a national study. *JAMA* [serial online]. 1998;279(19):1548-1553. Available from: Ovid Technologies, Inc. Accessed April 23, 2000.

Berman BM, Singh BB, Hartnoll SM, Singh BK, Reilly D. Primary care physicians and complementary-alternative medicine: training, attitudes, and practice patterns. *J Am Board Fam Pract* [serial online]. 1998;11(4):272-281. Available from: Ovid Technologies. Inc. Accessed June 3, 1999.

Bhattacharya B. MD programs in the United States with complementary and alternative medicine education opportunities: an ongoing listing. *J Altern Complement Med.* 2000;6(1):77-90.

Crock RD, Jarjoura D, Polen A, Rutecki GW. Confronting the communication gap between conventional and alternative medicine: a survey of physicians' attitudes. *Altern Ther Health Med.* 2000;5(2):61-66.

Devries JM. Emerging educational needs of an emerging discipline. *J Altern Complement Med.* 1999;5(3):269-271.

Eisenberg DM, Davis RB, Ettner SL, Appel S, Wilkey S, Van Rompay M, Kessler RC. Trends in alternative medicine use in the United States, 1990-1997: results of a follow-up national survey. *JAMA* [serial online]. 1998;280(18):1569-1575. Available from: Ovid Technologies, Inc. Accessed April 23, 2000.

Engebretson J. A heterodox model of healing. *Altern Ther Health Med.* March 1998;4(2):37-43.

Eskinazi D. Muehsam B. Factors that shape alternative medicine: the role of the alternative medicine research community. *Altern Ther Health Med.* January 2000;6(1):49-53.

Flores G. Culture and the patient-physician relationship: achieving cultural competency in health care [Invited commentary]. *J Pediatr* [serial online]. 2000;136(1):14-23. Available from: Ovid Technologies, Inc. Accessed April 27, 2000.

Hopwood AL. The social construction of illness and its implications for complementary and alternative medicine. *Complementary Ther.* 1997;5:152-155.

Hufford DJ. Culturally grounded review of research assumptions. *Altern Ther Health Med.* 1996;2(4):47-53.

Hufford DJ. Folk medicine and health culture in contemporary society [Review]. *Prim Care;* 1997;24(4):723-741.

Jobst KA, Shostak D, Whitehouse PJ. Diseases of Meaning, Manifestations of Health, and Metaphor [Editorial]. *J Altern Complement Med.* 1999;5(6):495-502.

Jobst KA. Obstacles to healing in medicine and science: the interplay of science, paradigm, and culture. *J Altern Complement Med.* 1999;5(5):391-394.

Kaptchuk TJ, Eisenberg DM. The persuasive appeal of alternative medicine [Perspective]. *Ann Intern Med* [serial online]. 1998;129(12):1061-1065. Available from: Ovid Technologies, Inc. Accessed April 23, 2000.

Kim C, Kwok YS. Navajo use of native healers [Original Investigation]. *Arch Intern Med* [serial online]. 1998;158(20):2245-2249. Available from: Ovid Technologies, Inc. Accessed April 23, 2000.

Kleinman A. *Patients and healers in the context of culture: An exploration of the borderland between anthropology, medicine, and psychiatry.* Berkely, California: University of California Press; 1980.

Millet S. Reflections on Traditional Medicine. *J Altern Complement Med.* 1999;5(2):203-205.

National Center for Complementary and Alternative Medicine. *NCCAM Strategic Plan to Address Racial and Ethnic Health Disparities.* Available at http://nccam.nih.gov/strategic/health_disparities.htm. Accessed August 3, 2001.

Owens JE, Taylor AG, Degood D. Complementary and alternative medicine and psychologic factors: toward an individual differences model of complementary and alternative medicine use and outcomes. *J Altern Complement Med.* 1999;5(6):529-541.

Pachter LM, Cloutier M, Bernstein BA. Ethnomedical (folk) remedies for childhood asthma in a mainland Puerto Rican community. *Arch Pediatr Adolesc Med.* 1995;149(9):982-988. Available from: Ovid Technologies, Inc. Accessed May 3, 2000.

Pachter LM, Sumner T, Fontan A, Sneed M, Bernstein BA. Home-based therapies for the common cold among European American and ethnic minority families: the interface between alternative/complementary and folk medicine. *Arch Pediatr Adolesc Med* [serial online]. 1998;152(11):1083-1088. Available from: Ovid Technologies, Inc. Accessed April 24, 2000.

Pachter LM. Culture and clinical care: folk illness beliefs and behaviors and their implications for health care delivery [Special Communication]. *JAMA* [serial online]. 1994;271(9):690-694. Available from: Ovid Technologies, Inc. Accessed May 3, 2000.

Risser A. Use of folk remedies in a Hispanic population. *Arch Pediatr Adolesc Med* [serial online]. 1995;149(9):978-981. Available from: Ovid Technologies, Inc. Accessed May 4, 2000.

Straus SE. Statement by Stephen E. Straus, MD, Director, National Center for complementary and Alternative Medicine before the Senate Appropriations Subcommittee on Labor, HHS, Education and Related Agencies on the Fiscal Year 2001 President's Budget Request for the NCCAM, Thursday, March 30, 2000. [National Center for Complementary and Alternative Medicine Web site]. Available at: http://nccam.nih.gov/nccam/ne/appropriations-s.html. Accessed April 3, 2000.

Straus SE. Statement by Stephen E. Straus, MD, Director, National Center for Complementary and Alternative Medicine before the Senate Appropriations Subcommittee on Labor, HHS, Education, and Related Agencies, March 28, 2000. [National Center for Complementary and Alternative Medicine Web site]. Available at: http://nccam.nih.gov/nccam/ne/senate.html. Accessed April 3, 2000.

Wynia MK, Eisenberg DM, Wilson IB. Physician-patient communication about complementary and alternative medical therapies: a survey of physicians caring for patients with human immunodeficiency virus infection. *J Altern Complement Med.* 1999;5(5):447-456.

INDEX